Pivot
to
Find
Your
Joy

Pivot

to

Find

Your

Joy

Joy Ohayia, PhD

iUniverse

PIVOT TO FIND YOUR JOY

Scripture quotations marked NKJV are taken from the New King James Version. Copyright © 1982 by Thomas Nelson, Inc. Used by permission. All rights reserved.

iUniverse books may be ordered through booksellers or by contacting:

iUniverse
1663 Liberty Drive
Bloomington, IN 47403
www.iuniverse.com
844-349-9409

ISBN: 978-1-6632-0753-1 (sc)
ISBN: 978-1-6632-0754-8 (e)

Library of Congress Control Number: 2020916134

Print information available on the last page.

iUniverse rev. date: 09/16/2020

I dedicate this book to People in Search of Finding Their Joy.

Be Blessed, Stay Healthy!

Contents

Acknowledgements

"I can do all things through Christ who strengthens ME."
Phil 4:13

To My Lord and Savior Jesus Christ, I am Forever Grateful.
Thank You!

To:

My Mother, Ruby
My Father's Spirit, Willie "Floyd"

My Husband, Partner in Love for Life Even as Ghosts, Chiji

My Sons, Chikezie and Kemji
My Daughters in Love, Rebecca and Naintara

My Brother, Nate

My Family and Friends

I love you, thank you for your support.

A Special Thank You

Joe Tartaglia – Cover design and interior illustrations.
Thank you, thank you, thank you for your creativity and patience.

Foreword

No better time for 'Pivot to Find Your Joy' than where we are right now,

During this Pandemic 2020 – we search for guidance, for love, to get through this crisis somehow,

Amidst the chaos and fear – behold a book with sage Wellness and Life ideas to see one through,

Whatever life throws at you,

I knew when I met Dr. Joy Ohayia that she was a force – determined to have a say,

Would not back down, would find a solution, somehow, some way,

Already a published author, a successful radio and television Host with degrees to show,

That on health and wellness and life, there was none other more in the know,

Plus an award-winning track and field star who rose above all those demands,

Her record, 3 decades later, remains unbroken and still stands,

A philosopher, an environmentalist, nutritionist and so spiritual – approachable and real,

She's a mathematical financial wizard – and knows the true art of the deal,

Intellectually astute, mentally sharp and emotionally tough,

Who bravely reveals her life when times were rough,

The Chapters ahead are each relevant and chock full of common sense for all,

Starts with Mental/Emotional Wellness - jam packed with relatable issues,

But I must warn you, before you sit down to read, get a box of tissues,

There's guidance on Nutrition – there's always something to teach,

Just the facts and examples, Dr. Joy does not preach,

Physical Wellness – explores the importance of self-love and self-care,

So many people neglect themselves or their needs – don't be one of them - don't you dare,

Where would we be without Social Wellness – really not too far along,

This chapter highlights the importance of connection – told mostly in song,

Intellectual Wellness – so important to stay sharp at any stage,

This Chapter offers ways to accomplish this at any age,

Financial Wellness is tricky even for those who have the tools,

This Chapter is a must read for anyone seeking advice on some 'not so well known' rules,

Environmental Wellness – so important for our planet and I must utter,

Please don't use plastic (ever) and it's important for our home (and brain) to de-clutter,

The Chapter on Spiritual Wellness explains drawing strength from the Source,

Whatever that means to you – it's personal, yet universal – of course,

This book has it all – plus it's inspiring and a quick read,

Engaging, informational, forth-coming – it has everything one might need,

Everyone faces a pivot in life, whether in love, relationships or employ,

Do it with grace and gratitude - 'Pivot to Find Your Joy'!

Amy Wachtel Delman, Poet

Health Disclaimer - Dr. Joy Ohayia, QuantumQuest LLC will not be held responsible for client injuries, allergies, and all dietary problems sustained due to consumption of food mentioned in this book. Food choices may vary due to individual responses. It is recommended you avoid foods that may cause you to have an allergic reaction. Medical clearance from your physician is recommended prior to embarking on a physical fitness routine.

Pivot to Find Your Joy –

A Call To Action for My Readers…

Introduction

What's Up Beautiful People?

The timing for this book could not come at a better time as the year 2020 is one for the history books - one of the most disruptive years in the twenty-first century, as COVID -19, the global pandemic and the exponential surge of protests against police brutality and for racial equality, had the world at a standstill and in disarray.

Recent studies have shown, 45% of Americans have reported that their mental health has been negatively impacted by COVID and whatever Joy we had was lost due to changes in the economy, increased unemployment, grieving lost loved ones, sheltering in place, sickness, lack of resources, healthcare disparities, bare shelves in the supermarket, stress, and riots, just to name a few.

Sunk in quarantine and uncertainty, we now belong to a new normal. An inexplicable fear and stress define our lives as we struggle to return to normalcy. Here's the deal, how we defined normal prior to COVID-19, is in our past, we have been forced to redefine our new normal. Did we lose our Joy in the process? You bet many of us did! So, now we have the opportunity to get it back.

When was the last time you felt JOY?

What is JOY? Merriam Webster defines Joy simply put, as a state of happiness.

"Pivot to Find Your Joy" is infused with my personal experiences (the good, the not so good, and the ugly), common sense approach with practical tips in the areas of Mental and Emotional, Nutritional, Physical, Social, Intellectual, Financial, Environmental and, Spiritual Wellness.

A CALL TO ACTION… to help you Pivot to Find Your Joy.

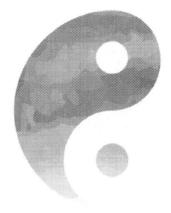

CHAPTER 1

Mental and Emotional Wellness

Mental/Emotional Wellness, according to the World Health Organization, is defined as "a state of well-being in which the individual realizes his or her own abilities, can cope with the normal stresses of life, can work productively and fruitfully, and is able to make a contribution to his or her community." Emotional wellness inspires self-care, relaxation, stress reduction and the development of inner strength.

My Story...

Yes, a stable mind. Along with stable emotions. You can never overestimate the value of keeping your emotions in check. What they say about the mind-body connection is so true. Our relationships and our self-esteem are two components that can alter our emotional wellness. *WARNING ALERT: If our mind is right, we can achieve anything – okay, most things.* You will never find peace of mind until you listen to your heart.

On that note, let's move forward. I started deep breathing exercises on a regular basis during my PhD studies back in 2007. Why? Because back then my middle name should have been *WORRY.* Yep, that was me – I worried all the time.

As a child, my parents were a positive force in the Universe and in my life. Their message to me was "Joy, always do your best", however at the age of 5, I began to hear and interpret the very same message "Joy, always do your best" as "Joy, Be Perfect". OMG! That's a lot for a little girl and even a grown woman to process. This is when the conflict began. Hence, I will say it again, my middle name from childhood to young adulthood, matter of fact right through my fourth decade (that would be through my forties) should have been *WORRY.* I had a lot going on in life and I wanted to make sure I got it right.

So, I tried to be perfect. With my grades, my relationships, my competition on the track *(well, okay, this was also for pleasure and a great outlet),* but still I focused on getting the "Wins" for the team and for me of course, a great self-esteem boost. Everyone should have *internal personal little things* to increase your own self-esteem. And I learned a very valuable lesson. Yeah, what's that? News Flash! There is NO One perfect.

Over the years, I have relaxed the idea of being perfect, of perfection in general, however; I always try to do *my best.* There is a difference.

It is important to not complain – just do...as there is always a solution to a perceived problem.

One of the ways I use to figure out a path when stuck is to turn negative statements in my head into positive thoughts. How? By practicing and using mantras. My favorite mantra is "I AM WHO I AM AND IT IS GREAT TO BE ME! I look at myself in the mirror each morning and state my mantra. This is my guide for the day – would you try it? Say it out loud or say it quietly – "I AM WHO I AM AND IT IS GREAT TO BE ME." Practice it. Soon it will become a habit. Soon, you will start to believe it. Soon, it will become reality. It feels really good and it is very healing and healthy.

I also believe in the importance of self-care. Body massages and pampering sessions in general are routine every two weeks, for me mentally and physically.

Equally important to me is the concept of *Authenticity* and *Core Beliefs*. "Are We Functioning Under Conflicting Knowledge Every Day"? I actually published this quick read in 2017 on Amazon. Here is a snippet "Thoughts are the basis of our internal processing, but they tend to cluster into what we call ideas, then an interesting thing happens; the ideas cluster again and become what we recognize as core beliefs and the whole process takes a left turn into *conflict land*. This conflict could potentially wreak havoc on our mental wellness. Authenticity is a quality we may seek, and it begs the question: Is this a state or something that we can achieve by will or is it just buried underneath a pile of conflicts trying to get out?

Can it be that it's tied up in thoughts we are thinking on a regular basis that are not congruent with our personal codes and cause us discomfort for which we seek escape? Is this a vicious cycle that so many of us in the modern world have seamlessly woven into our personal fabric and have come to accept as the way it is? Even if we see, acknowledge, and accept that our own internal processes hold us back from being more authentic; what is it that holds us back from choosing and experiencing the joy we profess to want? I fully believe that as the consciousness of a person is resolute to reducing internal conflict, their authentic self will emerge to promote *positive increased significance* in others."

Thankfully, I am not guided by the content on Social Media – as a matter of fact, every year for Lent (40 days), I suspend my social media activity. Ok, I answer email. But no active engagement on my social media feeds, Instagram, Twitter, and both FaceBook pages. It is sooooo liberating! A time for me to decompress. Isn't it interesting that you need to *disconnect virtually* in order to *connect in real life*? Connection is the true essence of living a full life. Our past experience confirms at every point that everything is linked together, everything is inseparable.

As I write this book, the entire world is experiencing the pandemic of COVID-19. We have been forced to lock down, to *shelter in place* and to adhere to *social distancing* when out and about. Never before have we had to *disconnect* so totally from life. Many of us have never experienced this type of forced retreat, unless you were alive when the Spanish Flu hit – that was back in the early 1900's. Highly doubt it! Yet, more than a hundred years ago, the world recovered, and we will too. It is hard to believe sometimes, when there is no clear path forward as of yet. This is where faith comes in. *Faith* is taking the first step even when you do not know what is going to happen next.

Here are a few things I did during the lock down:

I kept a positive attitude and only allowed myself to think healthy and productive thoughts. A mind that harbors negative thoughts usually causes its body to function in negative ways. Staying healthy and safe were my priority so my family followed the protocols that health organizations published. Yes, we wore face coverings when we left the house. Of course, we did! I kept my mind active. Hey, I am writing this book. Hello! Along the same lines, my body remained in motion, by doing alternating yoga, core, and stretching exercise workouts at home. You can do it too as there is no equipment necessary, just a floor and mat (optional). I was able to clear my mind for the upcoming daily activities - first and foremost, I did something for myself. Yep, I took care of ME.

As the pandemic wore on, I continued writing daily gratitude journal entries and praying daily for the health and safety of myself, family, extended family, friends, colleagues, acquaintances, first responders, anyone that was on the front line, and folks outside my circle. When the weather was nice, I would make an effort to spend at least 30 minutes outdoors soaking up the sun or through a brisk walk.

On a few occasions, I took a trip back into the past to reflect on good times and key learnings. This was indeed a most challenging time for everyone, not just Americans, this was a global pandemic. Going back to happier times will counterbalance all the bad news bombarding us 24/7. As I write this book in 2020, we have no idea when the pandemic will end or the state of our economy in the future. Heavy, right? Need a break for a while? Practice positivity. How? Start by reading this: *positive thinking changes the way we behave.* I believe that when I am positive, it not only makes me better, but it makes others around me better as well.

So, make everyone around you better. Connect with family and friends via phone conversations, text threads, FaceTime, Zoom, and Google Hangout, Google Duo. Hey, this is the good side of social media, use it for doing positive things!

Prior to the lockdown period, my husband and I had plans for international excursions to China, Italy, and Greece. Needless to say, those plans were halted. Now they are back on our *travel list* and hopefully we will get to visit and expand our cultural knowledge when it is safe to travel again. Our travel list is pretty long as there are 196 countries in the world, our goal is to see/experience as much of it as possible. So, a global pandemic can shake one to the core and everyone understands. We are all in the same boat. No shame as no one questions why you are so upset!

But life is full of other challenges – and you can be *shaken to the core* when some of these happen. The difference is, they do not appear as dangerous at first. They appear as friends. As loving friendships. Specifically, best friends. Uh oh!

When I met someone that I connected with *girlfriends*, looking back I would jump in 100%! That's how I roll. Yet, often I would find disappointment as I had expectations that were not always reciprocal. Through years of being hurt, I devised strategies on how to mitigate the risk of getting hurt.

My advice is to increase your spirit of discernment when it comes to *who* you choose to be in your inner circle. As a matter of fact, have several circles, as everyone does not deserve to be in your *front row.* Unfortunately, when relationships come about in various ways, there can be common interests that draw folks together. It is hard to discern the *balcony people* and the *good people* from the rest. They all dress the same. Trust is so hard to come by. This is the reason why my circle is small and tight, as tight as a dot, that's pretty darn tight!

I am now going to bear witness to a very painful period in my life. Talk about a strained long-term relationship OMG…there is soooo much drama with this one, I will spare you the details…oh, maybe not…here it goes…otherwise, how will you benefit from the lessons I learned?

This was a 25 + year relationship that waxed and waned over the years as we severed the relationship a few times then made attempts to rebuild. Talk about drama and stress – this became a tumultuous and pretty toxic time. However, and here' the rub: *I actually thought the relationship was good.* WOW! Why would you think that? Because. Whenever we took a break, I was told relationships take work. So, I would get to work. But how much work is productive? How much work should one dedicate to fixing something that just did not seem to want to get fixed?

In time, I thought this is too much, I do not go through this much *drama* with anyone else. I probably would not have put up with it for as long as I did with anyone else. She was a *girlfriend* – not a spouse, not a relative, but a *friend*! I trusted her and loved her. Deeply.

There was love on both sides as she considered me her sister as she often stated we were closer than her own siblings. I am an only child, at the time she was the closest I had to a sibling, we really clicked or so I thought. She had me at HELLO.

Then I began to notice something strange. There were threads of lack of support (as one would expect from a close sibling) whenever there was an achievement on my side. Hey, why did I feel then that I was going to throw up? I love her – why is my gut hurting so? I let it go, obviously over the years, then I began to reflect on our encounters over the last 10 years and I finally woke up and saw the blinding light of TRUTH! This was a one-sided relationship infused with some elements of disrespect.

This relationship created *nasty anxiety* as it was very tense. Confused, I continued with the relationship as we enjoyed many of the same things. However, something was not right, for years I did not feel at ease after our *getting* together. I began to really feel one should not have to work this hard for a sisterhood friendship, really! But I wanted her friendship.

Her actions were in my head – yep, subconsciously she was controlling my thoughts this was not a good thing. I would often ask myself what did I do? *Pay attention: should you experience this feeling in any relationship, it is a sign you are giving away your power.* Stop! Just Stop! Someone who truly loves you does not want power, they want you!

I gave as much as I could to the relationship, yet this was one sided at her convenience only. Then, again I began to reflect, I was not happy with the relationship for various reasons. I finally made the difficult decision to take the advice I have given to others over the years "*To take care of yourself mentally and emotionally, cut ties with people who hurt you.*" This relationship was causing me internal turmoil for a while. This was not good.

I finally I had to listen to my gut to preserve my mental and emotional wellness. This is paramount as your mind controls your actions!

I had to release myself from the relationship, at this point I could only *love* her and her family from a distance, which I mentioned to her at the time of our last meeting. We had our final meeting and it was tears on departure and painful from my side but very necessary. I was cutting ties with someone who hurt me deeply, most importantly, I was cutting ties with the *old* version of me, as I allowed that treatment to go on. I felt relieved the *nasty anxiety* was gone and I was a *better* version of me, with no regrets. But just in case you do have regrets in your own situations, remember your Mental/Emotional wellness is key to your mind/body connection. Your success. Your happiness. Yet, from time to time everyone feels afraid. Everyone. For times you start to feel that way; sit back and think positive thoughts.

You deserve it!

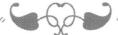

This was my mantra in 2010 and *still remains* a decade later.

"A Stable Mind is The Key to Total Wellness."
~ Dr. Joy

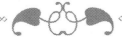

Here are some Mental and Emotional Wellness tips for you…

Let's begin the mental/emotional wellness section with Three Deep Breaths. Ready? Close your eyes, shoulders back with level head, breathe from your diaphragm to calm your frazzled nerves and cool your head, instantly.

On my count,
    Inhale...Exhale,
       Inhale...Exhale,
          Last one Inhale...Exhale.

Deep breathing.

Can be done anywhere at any time and is one of the best ways to lower stress in the body. Deep breathing: relieves pain, detoxifies the body, improves immunity, increases energy, lowers blood pressure, improves digestion, and helps support correct posture. When you breathe deeply, it sends a message to your brain to calm down and relax.

Imagine yourself at your own funeral.

Although this strategy is a little scary, it is effective at reminding us of what's most important in our lives. Question for you, when you look back on your life, will you be pleased at how uptight you were? Some wish they had spent more time with people they loved doing the activities they enjoyed. Imagining yourself at your own funeral allows you to look back at your life, while you still have the chance to make some important changes. While this is a bit scary, it is a good idea to consider your own death and, in the process your LIFE.

When you die, your "inbox" won't be empty.

So many of us live our lives as if the secret purpose is to somehow get everything done. We stay up late, we get up early, sometimes avoid having fun, and *we* keep our loved ones waiting. I used to do this myself. We convince ourselves that our *to-do* list is only temporary, and once the items are completed, we can then *rest*, have *fun*, and enjoy life. Here is reality, IT NEVER HAPPENS. Just as fast as the items are completed and crossed off the list, new ones appear. The nature of your *inbox* is that it is meant to have items, not to be empty. A full *inbox* is essential for success. It means your time is in demand, which is great!

Remember, nothing is more important than your own sense of happiness and inner peace. I too, must remind myself very often, that the purpose of life isn't to get it all done but to *enjoy* each step along the journey and live a life filled with happiness and love.

Do one thing at a time.

How often do we try to do more than one thing all at once? When we engage in multiple activities simultaneously, it is impossible to be present. Try this exercise: block out periods in time where you commit to doing only one thing at a time. Be present in *what* you are doing and concentrate. Two things may begin to happen:

1 – you may begin to enjoy what you are doing, even the mundane tasks, as when you are focused, rather than distracted, it enables you to become more absorbed and interested in the present activity; and

2 – you may experience an increase level of efficiency. It all starts with the decision to *do one thing at a time.*

Become more patient.

On a scale of one to ten, what is your patience level? Patience adds a dimension of ease and acceptance to your life. It is essential for inner peace. Becoming more patient involves opening your heart to the present moment, even if you don't like it. As your patience increases, you will become a more peaceful person and begin to enjoy the moments that caused frustration in the past. There is a reason for the delay. When a delay occurs, repeat the statement "This delay is good because…_____ "(fill in the blank).

A good cry is sometimes necessary.

Crying in healthy doses is a cathartic process that is healing, builds resilience and strength. I cry out of joy, sadness, grief, anger, fear, pain, and frustration. Better to cry than to hold it in.

Start a meditation practice.

There are scientific studies that show meditating helps to improve your mood, reduces stress, lessens anxiety, and increases your brain's grey matter, which is involved in muscle control, sensory perception, decision making, and self-control. In addition, once you get the hang of it, meditating is easy to do. For beginners, let's start:

1. Sit or lie comfortably.
2. Close your eyes.
3. Make no effort to control the breath; simply breathe naturally.
4. Focus your attention on the breath and on how the body moves with each inhalation and exhalation.
5. Length of time: Maybe try it for 1 minute in the morning. And when you can sit still and relax for that long, move to 2 minutes. Increase by 1minute increments until you reach 10 minutes per day. Focus on your breath.

Pick up a hobby.

Did you know that having a hobby is good for you? Hobbies can lower your stress levels, boost your brainpower, improve your ability to focus, and promote staying present.

Set aside one-hour-a-day to achieve your dreams.

Stop telling yourself that you simply do not have the time to work on your dreams. Whatever your dreams are, whether it is to make more money, learn to play an instrument, have a positive impact on the world, etc. if you devote one-hour-a-day to achieving your most important dream, by the end of the year you will have devoted 365 hours to that dream. Not bad!

Enjoy the little things.

Living life to the fullest doesn't just mean setting big goals it also includes learning to enjoy the little things, to appreciate life's simple pleasures, such as the following:

- Going outside at night to look at the stars
- Taking a walk outside
- People watch in a public place

Become more confident.

How is confidence defined? Confidence can be defined as your belief in your own abilities and in your capacity to get what you want. Confident people are happier, more relaxed, more likely to take chances, and more likely to succeed. To boost your confidence on a daily basis, give yourself credit for what you do, cultivate your inner advocate, and take consistent action toward the achievement of your goals. Watch your inner confidence SOAR!

Be kinder to yourself.

You may not be able to control how kind other people are to you, but you can always control how kind you are to yourself. Believe in yourself, respect yourself, and treat yourself well.

Create a positive attitude.

Having a positive attitude opens your mind to new possibilities, it makes you more resilient, and it can even help you to live longer. Your thoughts control your feelings, your feelings control your actions, and your actions control your results.

Minimize stress.

Stress – The Good, The Bad, and The Ugly. Did you know diseases are a result of uncontrolled stress and unhappiness? According to the CDC, heart disease is the leading cause of death for both men and women. About **610,000 people** die of heart disease in the United States every year, that's **1 in every 4 deaths**. For additional information, check out www.cdc.gov.

Here are some stress-less tips, referenced from *"Ohayia, J., Don't Let IT Get You", 2007 iUniverse* -

Love Yourself.
It is Ok to Say NO without feeling guilty. You are not a superhero.

Organize.
Use a daily planner to prioritize your tasks. This will give you a sense of control and reduce anxiety.

Treat Yourself.
Relax and Have Fun: Schedule massages, bubble baths and movie nights. Remember, FUN is individually defined.

Forgive.
Forgive YES, carrying a grudge, being envious or jealous of others, are destructive emotions because they require so much energy and may invite depression, guilt and shame. Let it go!

Let go of Worry.
You have NO room for negative thoughts. Worry is a wasted emotion that can affect your mental and physical health. More Faith Less Worry – 5 and 5, if it is not going to matter in 5 years, no need spending more

than 5 minutes thinking about it. "We don't get ulcers from what we eat, we get them from what's eating us."
~ Anonymous

Pivot in the direction of achieving "A Stable Mind" –

1) **Recharge your mindset.** Prolonged negativity lowers the immune response therefore increasing your risk of terminal illnesses. Think Positive Thoughts Daily! That's right every day, to increase YOUR self – esteem. Keeping in mind your positive thoughts will result in positive actions.

2) **Write down your positive thoughts.** Did you say you don't have pen or paper? Ok, well use your phone, as I know for sure it is in close proximity. Quit playing, many of you even name your phone, so now use it to scribe your positive thoughts using a Memo or Notes App. Remember only positive thoughts are allowed!

Smile.

Want to a simple, low cost way to reduce stress? Just smile. Smiling helps to generate more positive emotions within you." Say CHEESE…

Belly aching laughter.

Benefits of laughter (kid like) Chuckle even experience belly aching laughter. It is medically beneficial as laughter does wonders for your outlook. Research done by The Association for Applied and Therapeutic Humor, https://www.aath.org/ state children *laugh* more than 300 times *a day*, whereas adults *laugh* less than 20 times *a day*. Laughter is the best medicine as it heals a lot of hurts. Think about something that happened in the past that caused belly aching laughter.

Celebrate little victories.

Take a moment and pat yourself on the back. When you have attained your goal, whether little triumphs, small achievement, or life altering milestones. Self-praise is a nice way to remind yourself that you are making progress.

Apologize.

Do not let pride or ego get in the way, the words "I'm sorry", will make you feel better than the one to whom you are telling.

Walk Barefoot on The Beach.

When the weather permits…the beach has a way of sharpening all your senses while at the same time releasing tensions.

Vacation.

According to The Huffington Post, www.huffpost.com, a vacation or staycation will promote stress reduction, prevent heart disease, improve productivity, and increase peaceful sleep.

Surround yourself with people that push you to do better.

Seek to connect with people that focus on higher goals, increased motivation, good times, and positive energy to bring out the absolute best in each other. Quality people are more important than quantity. Back away from drama and negativity. No jealousy or hate. BLOCK it if you can.

Check-in with yourself multiple times a day.

How is your day going? Take a minute to check-in with yourself and figure out what you are focusing on. Are you stressed out because you are focused on the negative things that are happening? Or are you excited about the opportunities that are ahead of you? By intentionally bringing awareness to your thoughts and emotions, you can make a conscious decision to pivot your focus and interrupt the pattern of being on autopilot.

Check in With Others.

Here are 10 simple questions to choose from to ask when checking in on someone's mental health:

1) How are you feeling today, really? Physically and mentally.
2) What's taking up most of your headspace right now?
3) What was your last full meal? How much water have you consumed today?
4) How have you been sleeping?
5) What have you been doing for exercise? Yes the "E" word!
6) What did you do today that made you feel good?
7) What can you do today that would be good for you?
8) What are looking forward to in the next few days?
9) What can do together, even if we are apart?
10) What are you grateful for right now?

Perhaps lead off with question 10.

What is triggering your emotion?

Acknowledging negative thoughts and realizing that it's normal for your brain to be in reactive mode, gives you the power to make the conscious decision to pivot and focus on the opportunities instead of the problem. Be more aware of them instead of trying to fix them. Your emotions are not something you have to "fix." The trigger that made you feel that way is the thing to fix, not the emotion itself. By acknowledging you are not your thoughts, feelings and emotions, you become open to receiving the feedback and learning from them instead of reacting to them.

Win the battle in your mind before it becomes real.

Most of our fears and stressors are caused by what we think could happen. Much of the time, the fear isn't real, and only lives in our mind *False Evidence Appearing Real.* The thoughts of the worst-case scenario are all set in the future and are inspired by some pain from the past. Here is a secret weapon: you can win those battles in the same place, your mind. The BEST Strategy to combat fear is to learn to bring your attention back to the present. Practice keeping your attention on the *here* and *now.*

Increase your self-esteem.

How much you appreciate and like yourself? Your self-esteem is important because it heavily influences your choices and decisions. Take the quiz below to assess your self-esteem, check your score, and incorporate Dr. Joy's - Strategies for Achieving High Self-Esteem.

This is a quiz has been re-tooled and used during my health and wellness workshops and seminars, from The Rosenberg self-esteem test. The most commonly used measuring tool for self-esteem. A little history, it was designed in 1965 by Morris Rosenberg and is still being used today. Morris Rosenberg was a Professor of Sociology at the University of Maryland from 1975 until his death in 1992. He is known all over the world for his work on self-esteem and self-concept.

Quiz on YOUR self-esteem

A quiz for self-esteem is a way for you to determine how you see yourself. By being honest with yourself as to where you are today, you can see where you need to make improvements.

Your self-image is how you evaluate your own life, how you feel about your job, your relationships and where you are going.

How do you really feel about yourself? Do you have a harsh, negative opinion of yourself? Find out what kind of self-image you have by taking the quiz for self-esteem below.

For each question, choose one of the following answers. The number next to the answer represents how many points that answer is worth. Once completed, total your scores.

---

1 – Never 2 – Rarely 3 – Sometimes 4 – Usually 5 – Always

---

1. You express your opinions openly. _____
2. You have no fear of being rejected by other people. _____
3. When you have to make a major decision that affects mostly you (such as changing jobs), you may consult with other people, but the final decision is your own. _____
4. You forgive yourself for your mistakes. _____
5. You believe you deserve the best life has to offer. _____
6. You accept yourself for being the way you are. _____
7. You are able to express your feelings, both positive and negative. _____
8. You set aside some time just for you. _____
9. You ask for help when you need it. _____
10. You will return an unsatisfactory item to a store. _____
11. You don't worry about what others think of you. _____
12. If you are dissatisfied with an important part of your life, you will take steps to make a change. _____
13. You are comfortable making eye contact with other people. _____
14. When criticized, you listen, but don't take it personally. _____
15. You are comfortable trying new things. _____
16. You can make a list of your accomplishments and/or positive qualities without a great deal of difficulty. _____
17. You are comfortable around successful people. _____
18. You believe you can handle anything. _____

Your Total: _____

Remember, this is your current score. You have the ability to enhance your self-esteem. It begins with you!

Your quiz scores explained…

0 – 18: Time to Change - You question every decision you make and are crippled by lack of self-respect. Your self-esteem is dangerously low. You MUST make improving your self-esteem a #1 priority in your life.

19–36: Signs of Trouble -You believe other people are worth more than you are. Your self-esteem is shaky at best and needs work.

37-54: Middle of the Road -You have days when you think you're doing ok, and days when you question everything you do. Work on believing in yourself a little more, and everything will fall into place.

55-72: On the right track -Your faith in yourself is on the right track but can use improvement. Practice recognizing each small accomplishment and your self-esteem will start to soar.

73-90: Solid self-esteem -No one has to tell you that you're ok! You have a healthy sense of self-respect and rarely, if ever, question your decisions. You learn from your mistakes instead of dwelling on them. Keep up the good work!

Now that you have taken the quiz and tallied your results, here are **Dr. Joy's - Strategies for Achieving High Self-Esteem**

1) **Picture yourself succeeding.** Whatever challenge you are trying to face, work on believing that you will succeed. Being successful does not always happen with the first burst of effort. Imagine yourself attaining your goals and keep reminding yourself that you do not lose unless you quit.

2) **Love yourself.** Low self-esteem often comes about by being focused on the opinions of others. If you are looking for approval from someone else and they won't give it to you, you cannot win. Instead offer yourself love and approval no matter what, then you win no matter what the outcome of any given event.

3) **Work toward your goals.** If you want a better job but believe you cannot get one, you are right if you never get off the couch.

Instead if you send out a hundred resumes, you deserve self-respect just for making the effort. Break your goals into small steps that you can reach, such as sending out five or ten resumes a day. Be proud of yourself for each small step attained.

4) **Notice what you do right on a daily basis.** Each night before you go to bed, think about all of the things you did right that day. You can either do this on paper or mentally. This habit is one of the key methods of building high self-esteem.

5) **Learn from your mistakes.** A person with low self-esteem is crippled by their mistakes. Every mistake is an opportunity to learn something and to choose to do something differently the next time around. Make it a point to find the lesson in each loss and move on.

6) **Take time to do things you enjoy and perhaps learn something new.**

7) **Think positive.** Positive thoughts will result in Positive Actions and Results.

8) **Exercise.** Yes, I said the "E" Word.

9) **List five strengths you have.** Yes, I said YOUR Strengths... you have many, so start your list!

Take a break from social media.

How much time do you spend on social media on a daily basis? Be honest...1 hour, 2 hours, 3 hours or more a day? Social media, a force in today's society, has become an integral part of people's lives and daily routines. Many are addicted to it so much that is the first thing they do after waking up, is to check their social media. Get news highlights, share fun, interesting and informative content, engage with customers, and connect with people via social media can be a good thing, however there is a downside. The negative impacts of social media platforms include issues like increased levels of depression and anxiety, poor sleep quality, dissatisfaction with body image, decrease in self-esteem, cyber bullying, and FOMO (Fear of Missing Out). It is ok, to take a break.

Never ever compare.

Social media platform provides a catalyst for comparison, as we continue a cyclical habit of personal comparison from those around us. It goes like this: we observe others, we compare ourselves, we come up short, we feel bad, then to feel better we sharpen our observations, make more critical comparisons and ultimately feel worse. We reject our authentic self as a result we experience internal conflict. (Ohayia, J, Moore, G. *Are We Functioning Under Conflicting Knowledge Every Day?*, Amazon, 2017)

Be your authentic self.

Authenticity is not something we have but a goal. It is a work in progress and may take our entire lives to merge into that person, yet worth the effort.

Awaken your authenticity by:

Knowing thyself - a call to discover the true essence of your spiritual self.

Accept yourself – accept the *whole* you, your imperfections, strengths, weaknesses and insecurities.

Discarding the false self - the image of whom you think you are.

Do not associate with thoughts - thoughts come and go; yet the essence of whom you are is unchanging and authentic.

Be vulnerable – Open up. It is ok not to be perfect, as there is no "one" perfect.

Surrender addictions - let go of that which does not serve you, people habits, and things. Close the door and throw away the KEY.

Stop seeking validation - let go of the need to prove yourself to others. True validation comes from the core of your being.

Find time for silence – Just be still. Resolve to bring more peace by accepting what is, practicing non-judgment, and teaching your mind to become still.

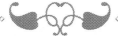

Who Are You Really?

Repeat: I AM WHO I AM AND IT'S GREAT TO BE ME!

You Are Who You Are …because everyone else is taken.

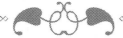

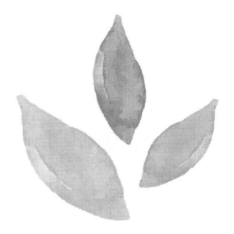

CHAPTER 2

Nutritional Wellness

Nutritional Wellness is an in-depth study of the nutrients our bodies need and how we can best provide those nutrients for optimal health and wellness. The course looks at government regulations regarding the safety of our food supply as well as technology in food production such as genetic modification.

My Story...

As a competitive athlete until 2008, guess what I was able to do? Yep, I was able to eat pretty much whatever I wanted. My workouts and my metabolism allowed me to eat my favorite foods without measure and still remain in great physical shape! Sorry, not sorry...okay, sorry! Some of my favorite foods, back in the day were chocolate desserts, pizza, pasta, grain bread, and, oh how I loved a good burger with bacon and cheddar cheese YUM! Are you still with me or did you turn the page? Spoiler alert – more favorite foods on the way - honey glazed carrots with white sugar and butter, fried salmon croquettes, oxtail stew, cornbread, pancakes with syrup or should I say syrup with pancakes, dough biscuits, sweet tea (OMG, sweet tea with my southern cuisine), fried chicken, French fries, and a good medium filet mignon steak. I think that just about covers everything! I knew this way of eating was not healthy nor sustainable as I was a heart attack ready to happen, but it was SOOO good. Hey, please don't judge. We all did crazy things in our younger years, right?

Check this out! I did not have any known food allergies; however, and this is where things start to change. On a trip to Martha's Vineyard, I had an 'out of body' experience (so very scary) after consuming calamari. I previously had a similar, much milder, episode during a business trip earlier in the year, but during this sunset dinner at Menemsha, Martha's Vineyard, the way I felt REALLY frightened me. This was a strong allergic reaction like no other. I had trouble breathing from internal hives, and guess what, I was DONE with calamari! *DONE, DONE, DONE.* Thank God I survived.

Flash forward do not judge me for my prior eating habits. With my running days now behind me and growing older, I was no longer able to eat everything I wanted. I had convinced myself that while my active lifestyle kept my blood pressure in check and allowed me to burn off calories, I knew deep down that this eating style could very well lead to a heart attack or worse. Oh, did I mention? I do *not* have a passion for food shopping or meal preparation, yet I enjoy eating healthy foods. Oy vey! (Yiddish word for "I'm up a creek without a paddle")

So, I made the major life decision to change my style of eating, not a diet, but an *eating lifestyle* kind of change. Today, I refrain from consuming RED meat and pork, when eaten my body feels different, perhaps to the long period to digest. Nevertheless, I no longer eat it. (But no pity party for me) because my favorite foods today consist of, get ready for it: greens, black beans, chopped spinach/kale salad with raw veggies, really yummy yes, seriously, nuts, seafood - not calamari for sure, fresh fruit as a snack or blended juice, a non-creamy dressing, tuna, and baked salmon. You know what, I feel really good! If I am bad, (and like Donna Summer said in her hit song, *Last Dance "when I'm bad, I'm so so bad"* please tell me you are old enough to remember Donna Summer), I will have lightly breaded, fried fish. Yes, I still enjoy my chocolate desserts. Also, I enjoy my red wine occasionally – hey, it's heart-healthy, right? I do drink in moderation due to the sulfates. I try not to consume too much bread – I said try.

And then there's the game-changer: water! I make sure to consume adequate/proper amounts of water daily. I will provide your calculation in the tips – so keep reading. For starters, I consume 8 oz of water each morning prior to beginning my workout to reduce the lactic acid in my muscles. I encourage you to do the same, as soon as you get up each morning drink plain water – room temperature is best.

I did not take vitamins until the pre-menopause phase, yes, I know the 'M' word. I experienced *warm flashes* that became constant and uncomfortable *hot flashes* and then there were the *night sweats* that would disrupt my sleep. With the ceiling fan blowing hard and one foot above the covers, this was the only way I could be comfortable. My wonderful husband was freezing, always under the blankets to keep warm. Hey, some of you have been there too, right? So, I began taking vitamins when a guest on my cable television show, The Dr. Joy Show, came to the rescue. Like a *Knightess in Shining Armor*, Dr. Erika Landau, a pediatrician in New York, has earned my forever gratefulness. She recommended a daily intake of the following cocktail not red wine, but really, just as effective: B-Complex, Vitamin D 50mcg, and Magnesium 500mg, and after 28 days I found relief. *Important Note: Always consult your physician for advice.* In addition, I have also added Fish Oil as a daily vitamin. I was always told it is best to eat your nutrients; however, when we fall short (and who among us doesn't) then these vitamins are essential. A shot (2 capfuls) of apple cider vinegar once per day in the morning has been a game changer as it aids in reducing belly fat – yes, the stubborn belly fat we all hate.

Again, consult with your physician prior to beginning a new vitamin regime.

I feel great, look great (did I just say that?) and I am healthy. Is there anything in this world more priceless than that?

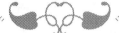

Everything in moderation.

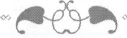

Here are some Nutritional Wellness tips for you…

Drink more clear water.

I know, I know, some of you are rolling your eyes... but we NEED water to LIVE. Our bodies are comprised of 70 + percent of water! We lose water daily, so we MUST be sure to replenish to keep our body healthy. Consume your proper amount of water daily to remain properly hydrated and lose/maintain your weight. Each day we lose water through sweat, urine and bowel movements. Even breathing uses water from our body. When you don't drink enough water, your energy will drop, and your mood will become more irritable. A dehydrated brain actually works much harder to achieve simple tasks, than when you are well hydrated. It even temporarily shrinks if you don't drink water.

Here is the deal about WATER - No additives: no lemon, no lime, no honey, nothing, just plain water.

1) The Best Source of Water is from fruits and vegetables also drink "pure" water daily to aid in food digestion and clean out the kidneys.

2) Simple Water Calculation: take your current weight and divide by 2 to get your recommended daily amount. Ex. 150lbs/2=75oz per day.

3) Is consuming too much water dangerous? Yes! To avoid water poisoning, do not consume more than 100 ounces per day.

4) Increase water consumption daily if you participate in strenuous activity, subjected to sun, wind, or high elevation to prevent dehydration.

5) Consume your water 5 times during the day: Upon awakening, 30 minutes prior to lunch, midday, after your workout, and 30 minutes prior to dinner.

6) Have trouble drinking from a cup or glass? Use a straw for ease of swallowing.

7) Avoid consumption of extreme water temperatures (Ice Cold), as this would hinder the digestive process. Room Temp is best!

8) Carry your water in a BPA free or stainless container for travel. I highly recommend investing in the LifeStraw Go 22oz.

Personal Water Bottle www.lifestraw.com. I love this bottle as it allows me to keep easy track of the amount of water consumed throughout the day.

Eat fewer calories.

Carrying excess weight puts us at a greater risk of a whole range of serious health problems, including heart disease, diabetes, and some cancers. Keep things simple. When you want to lose weight, eat less of the "comfort" foods and/or exercise to burn more calories.

Eat good food most of the time.

It is important that you enjoy what you are eating. Treat yourself to foods that taste good to you. Refrain from deprivation of your favorite foods as there is a chance of you becoming depressed. You already know, I love chocolate desserts, so I reserve the desserts for the weekend, a little treat to myself to celebrate a productive week.

Digestion, Digestion, Digestion…

A great question many ask, when should the heaviest meal be consumed? Here is the answer: during your lunchtime (in the middle of the day). Eating your heaviest meal during lunch time will allow longer digestion of heavy foods. It is also recommended to finish your last meal 2-3 hours prior to going to bed.

Apple cider vinegar.

Two capfuls (a shot) of apple cider vinegar alone or added to 8 oz. of plain water, will help with digestion and waste elimination. Be careful not to let the apple cider vinegar touch your teeth. Undiluted apple cider vinegar is acidic enough to weaken the enamel on your teeth, increasing your vulnerability to tooth decay and cavities, and cause your teeth to be sensitive.

Need a good snack.

If you are not allergic, eat a banana for a snack. Bananas are one of the world's finest foods for providing fuel for energy. Bananas contain a unique blend of vitamins, minerals and good carbs that foster a quick and efficient conversion to useable fuel. Leave the potato chips alone. I know sometimes this can be tough!

Eat more fruits and vegetables.

Your daily meal regime should include a variety in fruits and vegetables, which contain nutrients and phytonutrients to help prevent heart disease. Try to eat at least five servings of fruits and vegetables per day.

Eat nuts *(Only if you do not have an allergy).*

Nuts are rich sources of monounsaturated fats, which can lower cholesterol. Try one ounce of nuts per day including almonds, walnuts, peanuts, brazil nuts, and hazelnuts. If you are allergic to nuts there are good substitutes such as olives, pumpkin seeds, sunflower seeds and avocados are all excellent sources of monounsaturated fats.

Eat seafood *(Only if you do not have an allergy).*

Eating seafood once or twice a week increases the amount of healthy omega-3 fatty acids you eat and decreases your risk of heart disease. Fish such as mackerel, salmon, albacore tuna and sardines have the most omega-3 fatty acids. If you have a seafood allergy, flaxseeds, chia seeds, hemp seeds, soybeans and soy products will suffice.

Minimize consumption of red meat and pork.

Many love a good tasting steak, beef burger, sausage, or crispy bacon. Red meat, such as lamb, beef, pork and venison, is a rich source of iron and is important in preventing the condition anemia. Eating red meat once or twice a week can fit into a healthy meal regime. However, past research conducted by National Institutes of Health www.nih.gov, has tied red meat to increased risks of diabetes, cardiovascular disease and certain cancers.

For my readers that LOVE to read product labels, look for food stuff with monounsaturated fats.

Use monounsaturated fats.

Olive Oil and canola oil are high in monounsaturated fat, which help reduce blood cholesterol and may help raise HDL (the "good" cholesterol).

Increase your fiber.

Fiber helps lower cholesterol and people who eat more fiber have a lower risk for heart disease. Fiber is found in fruits, vegetables, grains, and legumes. Try to eat a minimum of 25 grams of fiber each day. Note: Be sure to check your allergies, in my case, oatmeal and I do not get along – my waistline expands instantly after consuming oatmeal = inflammation, therefore I stay away from oatmeal.

Reduce your sodium intake.

The human body only requires about 500 milligrams of sodium per day. Want to reduce high blood pressure? Try to cook without salt, with that said a great alternative would be vinegar and lemon juice as they stimulate some of the same sensory receptors as salt. My favorite no-salt seasoning blend is Mrs. Dash, it adds great flavor without the sodium.

Our bodies need vitamin D, but milk is a No No for our digestive system...

Here is the deal about milk...

It is the rule in nature that the young takes milk alone as milk is food for the young. Due to its protein and fat (cream) content, milk combines poorly with all foods as when it enters the stomach it will coagulate – form curds. Sounds nasty right? Wait, there is more... the curds may form around the particles of other food in the stomach insulating against the gastric juice – hence a strain on our digestive system. Still want dairy milk? Ok, try the following alternative plant-based options:

Coconut milk, Almond milk, Oat milk, Soymilk.

So, you have the question - what are great sources of vitamin D?

Very few foods in nature contain vitamin D. The flesh of fatty fish such as salmon, tuna, mackerel and fish liver oils are among the best sources. Small amounts of vitamin D are found in beef liver, cheese, and egg yolks.

For my Vegan readers, I've got you...beans and legumes can be a reasonable source of calcium, just keep in mind that you absorb about half of the calcium in beans that you would in milk. Eat more beans to make up the difference. Winged beans, soybeans, and white beans top the list of iron-rich beans.

Best way to cook your beans, plan ahead. One way you can get more calcium out of your beans is to soak them overnight in warm water. The process is simple, will reduce your cooking time, and will improve your ability to absorb the calcium in the beans.

Love to go out?

Not to worry, you can eat healthy while being social. Here are 20 healthy social eating tips from my first book, *"Don't Let "IT" Get You!"*

1) Order salad dressings and other sauces on the side to have control over how much or how little to add.
2) When ordering grilled fish or veggies, ask for grilled food without butter, oil. Here is another option, request prepared *light* with little oil or butter.

3) When ordering pasta dishes look for tomato-based sauces rather than cream-based sauces. Why, because tomato-based sauces are much lower in fat and calories. In addition, the tomato sauce or marinara sauce can count as a vegetable.

4) Drink water or unsweetened tea instead of regular soda or alcoholic beverages aka liquid empty calorie meals. This will reduce your calorie intake.

5) Share an appetizer and/or dessert with a friend. Half the dessert equals half the calories and half the price too. Don't want to share your dessert, check out healthy dessert options: sorbet, fresh berries or fruit.

6) Soup can serve as an appetizer or entrée. When choosing a soup, keep in mind that cream-based soups are higher in fat and calories than other soups.

7) Order steamed veggies as a side dish instead of starch.

8) Ask for salsa with a baked potato instead of sour cream, butter, cheese, or bacon. Salsa is very low in calories and a healthy alternative with a lot of spice!

9) Stop eating when full. Listen to the cues your body gives you. Do not feel obligated to stuff yourself.

10) Order sandwiches with mustard rather than mayonnaise or *special sauce*. Mustard adds flavor with virtually no calories.

11) Take half of your meal home. As a matter of fact, as soon as your food arrives, split in half and put in the *take-out* container. The second half will serve as a second meal.

12) To eat less, order two appetizers or an appetizer and a salad as your meal.

13) Side dishes? Opt for a baked potato or steamed veggies rather than French fries, I know it is hard. If you must have fries, try sweet potato fries, they are delicious. If choices are not listed, still ask your server to substitute veggies or baked potato instead of the French fries.

14) Baked, grilled, dry-sautéed, broiled, poached, or steamed. These cooking techniques use less fat in the food preparation and are generally lower in calories.

15) The restaurant industry is one of hospitality and customer choice. Dooooo not be afraid to ask for special low-calorie or low-fat preparation of a menu item.

16) Reduce bread in-take. I know it tastes so good. Ok, have your bread but without butter, letting go of the fat and calories.

17) Choose entrees with fruits and veggies as key ingredients. Enjoy the flavors they offer. Fruits and veggies are a good source of dietary fiber, vitamins, and minerals.

18) Choose foods made with whole grains. Whole-wheat bread and *love* the brown rice. When it comes to foods, *WHITE* is not right!

19) Herbs add a unique flavor to any dish. Try foods flavored with fresh herbs rather than fats such as oil and butter.

20) Downsize that Dinner. Many restaurants offer lunch sized portions of their dishes, which are smaller than their full-sized dinner entrees. Ask for the lunch portion as you will save your waistline some inches and your wallet some bucks.

Learn and remember the standards.

Three ounces of meat is the size of a deck of cards; 1 ounce of meat is the size of a matchbook; 1 cup of potatoes, rice or pasta looks like a tennis ball.

Last but not least, *Diets Fail Us*.

Enough Said! Up, down, up, down like a yoyo causes confusion to our bodies. Many of us want a quick fix, just remember, it took time to pile on the extra pounds, so allow time to lose the weight. Healthy Weight loss = One (1) – two (2) pounds each week.

Once you get to your desired weight, return to the beginning of the tips to ensure proper weight management. You can do it!

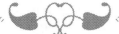

We Are What We Eat.

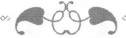

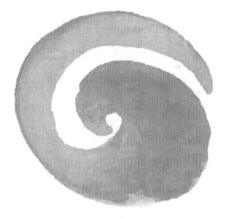

CHAPTER 3

Physical Wellness

Physical wellness is the ability to maintain a healthy quality of life that allows us to get the most out of our daily activities without undue fatigue or physical stress. Physical wellness promotes proper care of our bodies for optimal health and functioning. There are many elements of physical wellness that all must be cared for together. Overall physical wellness encourages the balance of physical activity, nutrition and mental well-being to keep your body in top condition.

My Story…

For most of us, our bodies change with time. No big secret there. I remember long ago when I was in my 20s and 30s, I believed I was going to be able to run forever. You see, running competitively was my thing! I was a Nationally ranked sprinter back in college with 3 individual records, one still remains unbroken to this very day in 2020, plus 1 relay record. Boy, I was fast. I was a member of two AT&T Corporate Running Teams. Extra bonus; I was able to travel to different parts of the country on the company's dime.

Now, a little bit of fantasy enters my story. After the birth of my sons, I was determined to keep in shape. As someone with a Mesomorph body type (a what?) *Important note: people with a mesomorph body type tend to have a medium frame.* We may develop muscles easily and have more muscle than fat on our bodies and we are typically strong and solid, not overweight or underweight. What a lucky girl I am, I was going to be able to stay in shape, the cardio would keep me in optimal condition for competition, not to mention looking fabulous! Dream on…Sleeping Beauty…dream on!

Reality bites! So, what happened? Well, I became pregnant with my older son. Due to complications, I almost lost him three times during the pregnancy, so I was forced to remain at home all during my last trimester. What did I do to pass the time? You guessed it, all I did was eat, my food and your food, too, if you took too long to finish what was on your plate. I gained 65 pounds during this pregnancy and our first son was born three days early. Whew! He was healthy, thank God!

Then came the second pregnancy which was completely different from the first go around. I worked until my 36th week, gained 70 pounds and our second son was almost 2 weeks late. But again, healthy, thank God! Boy, it was hot as hell in July 1993! After giving birth through c-section twice, I was able to lose the weight in both instances, a total of 135 pounds over three and half years – mind you! I was left with stubborn loose skin around my abdomen accompanied with less than tight abs and I hated it! Didn't just hate it – I HATED IT! I did not like to look at myself in the mirror, where did my sprinter body go?

Where were my tight abs and flat stomach? I worked out like crazy but the foopa was still there and not going away.

So, here's where the fairy godmother stops by for a visit. *(Hey, it's my story and if I want a fairy godmother – then I get one)* One day a friend of mine shared her secret to getting her body back. She showed me her flat stomach and mentioned it involved two things I feared the most – needles and knives. Yes, I have a *fear* of both. The answer was a tummy tuck with liposuction! I got over my fears - it was the best decision I made for myself, Thank You Dr. Carlos Burnett, Board Certified Plastic Surgeon - My internal confidence soared past the stars! Yes, I had plastic surgery to get rid of the loose skin, tighten my muscles lost during the c-sections, and most of all made me feel great about myself.

I continued to run and workout 5 days per week *(Yes, you heard that right)* during anytime I could get it in, sometimes in the morning while the kids were asleep, during lunchtime, or in the evenings during our sons Tae Kwon Do class. This was my outlet, my *me time*, plus I was taking care of the hardest working muscle in the body, my heart.

Still, I ceased competition in 2008 at the young age of 45. While staying in shape was essential; my competing priorities in *life* did not leave much time to train consistently for competitions. As mentioned before, running *was* my thing, until September 30, 2011. I remember it like it was yesterday. My husband and I were experiencing the empty nester pleasures for about 1 month as both of our sons were away at college – freeeeeedommmmm. I completed two workouts that day which consisted of a three-mile run and a short strength training session in our home gym. Being very ambitious, I decided to clear out the cabinets in our kitchen and plant mums in huge pots for our front door and on our driveway.

And then... And then what? *This is when my life began to change.* As I was bending and lifting the huge pots, I heard a pop…yet I kept going… *VERY IMPORTANT NOTE HERE – WHEN YOU HEAR A POP – STOP WHAT YOU ARE DOING – IMMEDIATELY!* Well, that pop ended my *normal running workouts* and since then I have never been able to experience the euphoric accomplishment, I get from running on a consistent basis (4-5 times per week).

So, what happened next? Glad you asked. Physical therapy pre and post-surgery was required and again no running. Recommended by my team of healers, was to forgo running and focus on core strengthening. Still terrified of needles and knives, my attempt to mitigate the pain was through physical therapy sessions. My new fear – paralysis! After months of physical therapy without relief, I succumbed to the idea of back surgery.

On July 19, 2012 (the day after our 25th wedding anniversary), I had a discectomy (L4-L5) region. Fortunately, no fusion! My orthopedic surgeon mentioned because I was in great physical shape, my surgery would be without complication and my healing process if I followed instructions (not usually my strong point) would take some time but I would resume to my normal activity level within 6 -8 months.

First few months were the toughest, as it was painful to walk around the block. Me, a sprinter, I now had to push past the pain just to walk around the block. Life does have an interesting way to teach us important lessons! I had to be patient – however *patience* is NOT in my vocabulary – sprinters move *fast* – they do everything *fast*. But I couldn't, so I didn't.

Post-surgery physical therapy sessions, time, patience along with positive thinking *eventually* led me to full physical recovery. Eleven (11) months post-surgery, I was fully recovered without drugs, no back pain and I began to slowly ease into getting back in shape through running on the treadmill. I had to take it slow and build back up speed and distance.

This experience taught me more about my body and sheer grit than anything I had been through before, and it is a lesson that continues to serve me well. Today, stretching, core workouts, and light yoga are part of my daily routine. That competitive *running* thing and USATF Masters World Ranking goal is only a dream, it will never happen. That dream died September 2011, however, as I have learned in life, when one dream dies, another is born. Today, I am living that dream: I am able to enjoy LIFE independently!

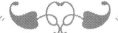

Your health is your wealth!

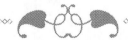

Here are some Physical Wellness tips for you…

Let's begin the physical wellness section with Three Deep Breaths. Ready? Close your eyes, shoulders back with level head, breathe from your diaphragm to calm your frazzled nerves and cool your head, instantly.

On my count,
    Inhale…Exhale,
        Inhale…Exhale,
            last one Inhale…Exhale.

Deep breathing.

Can be done anywhere at any time and is one of the best ways to lower stress in the body. Deep breathing: relieves pain, detoxifies the body, improves immunity, increases energy, lowers blood pressure, improves digestion, and helps support correct posture. When you breathe deeply, it sends a message to your brain to calm down and relax.

Get your eyes checked!

Dr. Kerry Gelb, OD of "Open Your Eyes Documentary" where he travels around the world and urges everyone to get our eyes examined. The optometric test of the eye is the easiest way to detect diseases in the body such as obesity, diabetes and Alzheimer's. For more information, check out - https://openyoureyes2020.com/.

Spend more time in nature.

We as humans are not made to be cooped up inside all day. Want to increase your happiness on a daily basis? Increase your creativity? If your answer is yes, then spend time in nature.

Move more.

It doesn't matter what you choose to do: join a sports team; get a pedometer and take at least 10,000 steps a day; get up every 20 minutes and stretch; or join a dance class. Just move! Living a sedentary life dumbs you down, it makes it more likely that you'll be overweight, and it puts you at a higher risk of depression.

Reduce lactic acid.

Consume 8 oz. of room temperature water, prior to beginning your workout, to reduce lactic acid in your muscles.

Exercise.

Yes, I said the E word! Exercise, no prescription required, it's free, it's legal, and it will give the glow of well-being!

Walking is great for relieving stress. Get up, move away from your desk and take a 10-minute walk outside – Refresh and soak up Vitamin D and clear your head.

Exercise has psychological and physical benefits as endorphins (chemical) released by your brain while exercising. Set your body in motion and let the oxygen cleanse your brain and clear away the cobwebs.

When is the best time to exercise? Morning if your schedule permits. Why? Because exercising early in the morning "jump starts" your metabolism, keeping it elevated for hours, sometimes for up to 24 hours! As a result, you'll be burning more calories all day long—just because you exercised in the morning. Also, exercising in the morning energizes you for the day—not to mention that gratifying feeling of virtue you have knowing you've done something disciplined and good for you. Yes, as it is all about YOU!

Wait, I know some of you are thinking, the "morning thing" does not work, no excuse, get in your daily exercise routine when your schedule permits. If the morning does not work for you, perhaps you are able to set aside time during lunch or after work.

Practice safety measures ALWAYS and listen to your body! Do not continue to exercise with an injury!

Consistent workout routines.

We have shared tips and benefits to get it moving and exercise daily. For my readers that have a desire to begin a consistent workout regime for a minimum of three days per week, Congratulations!

The first step is getting clearance from your physician. The second step is to determine your body type.

Some of you may wonder, what does your body type have to do with your workout? The answer: EVERYTHING! It is important, as one of your goals is to achieve optimal fitness. You are born into a body type and my recommendation to you is to accept *your body* and work consistently to make it healthier regardless of type.

Before, I go any further; I must state no one body type is greater, better, less than, or worse than the other. You cannot change your body type, as your bone structure will not allow such a change. By knowing your body type, you are able to understand your body, including why weight gain occurs in certain areas, experience difficulty gaining muscle/weight, or how to split your time between cardio and muscle toning to gain desired results.

No matter your age, your body type, YOUR ultimate goal is to achieve and maintain a healthy lifestyle.

Do you know your body type? Did you know that your body type determines your type of workout for you to yield optimal results? If you answered, YES to these questions GREAT…if not, that's ok…read on to get the information you need…

There are three broad body types:

Are You Ectomorph?

Slim body types that are linear in shape with narrow hips, short upper bodies, and long arms and legs.

Here are some facts about Ectomorphs:

1) You have a fast metabolism - you burn calories even resting,

2) Most likely very flexible,
3) You have very high endurance (sign of strong cardiovascular system),
4) You are unable to gain weight and muscle definition, and
5) With a thin physique, made of small bones and joints, you are more vulnerable to injury during extracurricular activities.

Common Myths about Ectomorphs –

You can eat anything and not gain an ounce. This is FALSE, as fat will build inside your body without proper care.

Note: THIN DOES NOT = HEALTHY! Don't Get IT Twisted!

Suggested Workout for Ectomorphs:

Muscle Strength and Conditioning = 60% of total workout time
Cardiovascular Activity = 40% of total workout time

Are You a Mesomorph?

This is a muscular body with thick bones. Muscles are tight and well defined: abs, thighs, gluteus, and calves…POW! This is ME.

Here are some facts about Mesomorphs:

1) Natural athletic build,
2) Full of energy and extremely competitive,
3) Ability to gain muscle easily and this will help protect the skeletal frame through the aging process,
4) Risk for obesity without proper nutrition and consistent exercise,
5) Greatest health threat: Cardiovascular disease,
6) Gains fat easily in the areas not so desired, might I add, and
7) Heavier appearance than actual due to your thick bones and muscles.

Suggested Workout for Mesomorphs:

Muscle Strength and Conditioning = 40% of total workout time
Cardiovascular Activity = 60% of total workout time

If you are thinking this body type sounds familiar, but you do not meet all of the criteria, relax there is nothing wrong with your DNA! The mesomorph body type has two sub-groups:

Meso-Ecto: Smaller bone frame but resemble the muscle size and build of mesomorphs. Meso-ectos also have a tendency to be lean, similar to the ectomorph, yet their natural strength is greater than that of the ectomorph.

Meso-Ecto Workout:
Muscle Strength and Conditioning = 50% of total workout time
Cardiovascular Activity = 50% of total workout time

Here is an example – if your schedule allows you to work out for one hour the days per week (Monday, Wednesday, Friday), you need to balance your routine to include equal amounts of cardio and muscle toning exercises.

Meso-Endo: Ability to gain a great deal of muscle mass, however vulnerable to extra unevenly distributed fat. To combat the extra fat, allot days and times for cardio exercises to stabilize a healthy body weight.

Meso-Endo Workout:
Muscle Strength and Conditioning = 40% of total workout time
Cardiovascular Activity = 60% of total workout time

Are you an Endomorph?

WOW! If you are an endomorph, you have a curvaceous body.

Here are some facts about Endomorphs:

1) Body fat settles into the lower regions of your body, predominately lower abdomen, hips, and thighs,
2) Small to medium bones, limbs are shorter in relation to the torso and musculature that is not well defined,
3) Resembles hourglass body type, and
4) Face higher inclination towards obesity.

Suggested Workout for Endomorphs:

Muscle Strength and Conditioning = 30% of total workout time
Cardiovascular Activity = 70% of total workout time

To lose excess body fat, include low impact cardio such as walking, swimming (if you like the water – swimming exercises every muscle in the body), and rollerblading.

Bottom line - more cardio less weights on upper body muscle toning.

Benefits of stretching anytime, anywhere.

So…when was the last time you stretched YOUR body? Honestly, during my younger days, stretching was not my favorite part of the workout, but as I *celebrate more birthdays*, it is necessary for me to stretch each day to remain flexible, balanced, keep great posture, and most of all prevent injury.

How to Stretch:

Target major muscle groups.
When you are stretching, focus on your calves, thighs, hips, lower back, neck and shoulders. Also stretch

muscles and joints that you routinely use at work or play.

Warm up first.
Stretching muscles when they are cold increases your risk of injury, including pulled muscles. Warm up by walking while gently pumping your arms or do a favorite exercise at low intensity for five minutes.

Hold each stretch for at least 30 seconds.
It takes time to lengthen tissues safely. Hold your stretches for at least 30 seconds — and up to 60 seconds for a really tight muscle or problem area.

Do not bounce.
Bouncing as you stretch can cause small tears in the muscle. These tears leave scar tissue as the muscle heals, which tightens the muscle even further — making you less flexible and more prone to pain.

Focus on a pain-free stretch.
Expect to feel tension while you are stretching. If it hurts, you have gone too far. Back off to the point where you do not feel any pain, then hold the stretch. STOP if it hurts!

Relax and breathe freely. Do not hold your breath while you're stretching. Let IT Go!

If you have a chronic condition or an injury, seek advice from a professional to prevent further injury. Most of all be patient with yourself as you recover.

Massage therapy (body work).
The most common place on the body for knots is in the neck and shoulder area. Treat yourself to a massage to

loosen the knots. It is therapy for your body and mind. Your body will be limber and your mind will follow. You deserve it!

Pray and plank every day.
Also, mentioned in Chapter 8 - Spiritual Wellness, doing plank exercises every day is a great way to strengthen your core. If we want to be specific, the plank strengthens the abdominals, back and shoulders. Pray and plank demonstration during a Women's Empowerment Workshop.

Here are instructions on "how to" plank:

1) Find a space on the floor (a flat surface). Use a mat or towel for extra cushion if needed. Loose fitting clothing.
2) Lay flat on the floor.
3) Raise your body on your forearms and toes. Keep your head down.
4) First time planking, it is most important to hold and keep your balance.
5) Hold your plank for 1 minute (yes, set your timer).
6) Plank daily, increase time by 30 seconds, each month.

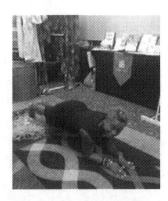

Go to bed.

Our body is like a battery; the only way to naturally recharge our body is to get enough REST! Small problems seem gigantic when you are tired. When you get adequate rest, you will feel refreshed and rested – you will feel that all things are possible.

So, how much sleep is needed? Continuous 7 - 8 hours of peaceful sleep. Now for the advice to get your rest…

If you feel sleepy during the day, go ahead and take a *cat nap*. Cat naps are no longer than 15 minutes. Close your eyes and ears to light and sound around you. This means, no phone, no watch, no tv, no radio, no laptop (on the lap on/near the bed). Try using ear plugs and/ or eye mask, I know for a fact this works!

Go to bed earlier, perhaps try 15 minutes earlier, or 30 minutes earlier and sleep. Just *shut it down*…until the act of sleeping is pleasurable. Again, as some of you did not get it the first time…no phone, no watch, no tv, no radio, no laptop on the lap on/near the bed.

Check this out, according to John Hopkins Medicine, engaging in physically active or demanding exercise means that your body needs *extra time* in bed. To improve your strength, endurance and speed you will need between 20% - 40% more sleep. So, here is the calculation: if you are getting 6 hours of peaceful sleep normally, increase your rest by 1 hour. Without the glaring light from electronics, switch your phone display to dark in the evening (beginning at 8 pm).

Are you able to awaken refreshed without an alarm clock? If yes, then your body is adequately recharged and ready to go.

Adopt a pet (Dog).

Dogs will force you to get up and get moving at least 3 times a day. Pets accept you for who YOU are. Our toy poodle Chipper shows us unconditional LOVE! Medical studies show that stroking dogs or cats lower blood pressure and brings a sense of peace. Chipper loves to be close to us and stroked – he never gets enough.

Have lots of safe sex.

Accomplish three things at once it melts, relaxes, and soothes. Did you know, each act burns on average 100 calories? The Men's Health study www.menshealth.com, found that on average, women burned about 69 calories for a 25-minute session, while men burned around 100 calories. According to experts, the key to high-calorie-burning sex is to make it hot and long. Enjoy!

Stand tall.

Walk with your head up, chest out, and shoulders back. An erect posture will aid in increased confidence and self-esteem. From a physical perspective, your breathing capacity increases, more oxygen rushes to your brain, and you are able to think more clearly.

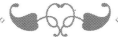

Repeat after me:
My Body is My Masterpiece!

I AM WHO I AM AND IT IS GREAT TO BE ME!

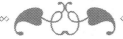

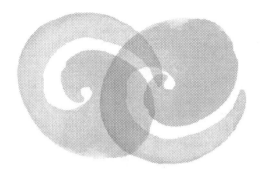

CHAPTER 4

Social Wellness

Social wellness refers to the relationships we have and how we interact with others. Our relationships can offer support during difficult times. Social wellness involves building healthy, nurturing and supportive relationships as well as fostering a genuine connection with those around you.

My Story...

Since my 20's, I thought I had many friends, all three phones (cell, home, and work) rang constantly until June 2005. Why? Because. When I was laid off from my financial services executive level position people stopped calling. Oh, no - who was calling in the first place? Friends or people that cared about Joy, or so I thought. Sadly, I was mistaken, most of the people calling during the time before June 2005 either needed or wanted a favor from me, and for some reason. Due to my lack of spirit of discernment, naivete, natural empathy, etc., I gladly helped the folks that reached out. Here's the thing though, back then I wasn't the type to complain *still true today* or ask for help, however, today *when necessary,* I gladly ask for help without reservation. I thought I had many friends until that fateful release from corporate bondage day in June 2005. Wow, did that hurt!! Let's listen to what Camilla Cabello had to say about finding out your friends may not be your friends in her song, 'Real Friends'.

> *Real Friends*
> *I'm just lookin' for some real friends,*
> *All they ever do is let me down,*
> *Every time I let somebody in,*
> *Then I find out what they're all about,*
> *I'm just lookin' for some real friends,*
> *Wonder where they're all hidin' out,*
> *I'm just lookin' for some real friends,*
> *Gotta get up out of this town!*

Camilla hit the nail right on the head with that one! I remember that day as if it was yesterday. Once being told, "effective immediately, your job has been terminated", I called my husband to give him the news. He asked, "how are you feeling?", then followed with "take the summer off and figure out what you want to do, I will support you", fast forward, he has kept his promise as I write this book in 2020 during the "shelter in place" and social distancing mandate – from 2005 – 2020,

15 years! And still counting. Luckily, it did not take me long to find my passion. I began my entrepreneurial journey immediately after being given my separation papers from corporate America. With my husband by my side, I knew we were going to be alright. Or as Switchfoot sang;

> *It's okay to feel,*
> *To say all the things you've been trying to hide,*
> *Lift it up to the ceiling,*
> *'Cause we all need that healing,*
> *Let's get lost in the feeling, the feeling,*
> *The feeling,*
> *We're gonna be alright!*

And eventually I was! For the next two years my social interaction with people changed as my focus shifted from working in corporate America to embarking on my entrepreneurial journey. Did I have unconscious expectations of the people in my circle? I certainly did, again, out of sheer lack of comprehension that frenemies can camouflage very well as friends when it suited them! By the way, I lumped everyone into one circle prior to June 2005. Yes, and that's the main reason for my hard lesson of disappointment. You all know what I'm talking about, right? Well, in case you don't – here's a little reminder;

> *We Used To Be Friends*
> *A long time ago*
> *We used to be friends*
> *But I haven't thought of you lately at all*
> *If ever again*
> *A greeting I send to you*
> *Short and sweet to the soul I intend – The Dandy Warhols*

The first year of entrepreneurship, was tough, as my focus was GOD, family, then business. My circle of self-employed/people in business grew. One lesson, I realized, is that not everyone that smiles in your face is happy for you. Oh, no, they are surely not, trust me. I began to foster new relationships – glad I did. Someone will ask – have the folks returned from pre-layoff back in your circle? Answer: Some are, however not in the inner circle. My inner circle is precious, you just don't get a pass in, it has to be earned! Like these people are never, ever getting back in – Oh, who?

> *The Backstabbers*
> *What they do?*
> *They smile in your face*
> *All the time they want to take your place*
> *The back stabbers (Back stabbers) - The O'Jays*

Since then, I have pretty much categorized folks: Family, Friends, Acquaintances, and Tangent Circle Members folks (which means the previous relationship has been severed, probably over some bullshit for which I do not have the bandwidth to endure - I will love you from a distance, no hard feelings). Carrying a grudge is not worth it! A good supportive person is vital to success in every aspect of your life. True friendship *in my opinion* should never be toxic nor hurtful. Sometimes, it is very, very hard to see which relationships are toxic. I think the group Green Day capsulized it perfectly in their song 'Good Riddance', don't you agree?

> *Good Riddance (Time Of Your Life)*
> *Another turning point, a fork stuck in the road,*
> *Time grabs you by the wrist, directs you where to go,*
> *So make the best of this test and don't ask why,*
> *It's not a question, but a lesson learned in time,*

So important to foster nurturing relationships. Surround yourself with positive people who will support you when you need advice and perspective. Friends should ADD to your life not take away; if someone is too exhausting or drains too much energy from you, take a break from that person until you have the available emotional fortitude. Sometimes the break may be permanent. The Beatles knew the importance of having good friends who are with you through everything – the good, the bad, the not so good, etc.

> *With A Little Help From My Friends*
> *What would you think if I sang out of tune?*
> *Would you stand up and walk out on me?*
> *Lend me your ears and I'll sing you a song,*
> *And I'll try not to sing out of key,*
> *Oh, I get by with a little help from my friends,*
> *Mm, I get high with a little help from my friends,*
> *Mm, gonna try with a little help from my friends,*

I was an only child in a two-parent household and grew up in Bronx, New York. The school I attended was Our Saviour Lutheran School from K-12. Yep, I was a lifer! I was bullied as a child in the South Bronx neighborhood as I did not have any back up, through middle school until we moved to the North Bronx. I can still remember that day, as I was thrilled beyond measure. I did not have the physical strength to fight back, so I obsessed with being perfect, doing the right thing, staying out of trouble. As I matured, I realized no one is perfect and there is no one perfect! I always enjoy meeting new people, sharing experiences, learning something new, keeping it positive! This is what I was born into, went through and survived and thrived.

Interestingly I had more male friends than female friends growing up. I made long lasting friendships/connections with several high school classmates and we are still in touch since 1975! Equally as important are my two college BFF's that I have had since 1980. Our marathon conversations, just catching up without judgment are the BEST.

Initially, I put friends in the same bucket - 1 big bucket. It was not until June 2005 when the change occurred, which is a shame, because I would give the shirt off my back for the people I love. *Their loss – oh well.* I love to share knowledge with others and travel is a huge part of my life and learning. I traveled with my parents as a young child and just love the new experiences, new cultures, everything! Luckily, my husband shares this passion!

Slowly, I started to care less and less about fitting in during my 30s and it increased each decade and by 50, my mindset has been "I SO Don't Care!" And when you really don't care, new doors begin to open.

In 2010, I became Producer and Host of the award-winning local cable TV show – "The Dr. Joy Show – Your Prescription For Total Wellness", with a focus physical, nutritional, social, environmental, financial, spiritual, and emotional/mental aspects. I began working with an Acting Coach to increase my skills and confidence with work on tv, stage, and film.

From 2013 – 2017, I served two terms, as a Board Trustee for the State of New Jersey chapter of CASA, a children's advocacy group, I was cast in the Off-Broadway play, 'Casey 30 Years Later' where I had four roles including the role of Dr. Joy. 2017 saw me named Mrs. Central New Jersey, and then in 2018, Mrs. New Jersey America Pageant where I met many people during this process. Check this out, this is something I would have not thought of – I was not a pageant girl.

Not too long after, I became Producer and Host of the "The Joy of Living" radio show - broadcasting on the dial of 920 AM The Jersey Fox Sports Radio. This show offered a parachute for radio listeners, providing relatable wellness experiences to find and embrace their Joy. Remember: We All have tremendous POWER – We Need to Use It.

One of my favorite books is "*The Four Agreements*" by Don Miguel Ruiz, gifted to me when I was laid off. I was forced to reflect and make changes as necessary. Fostering Nurturing relationships – For me Improving on My Spirit of Discernment (Don Miguel Ruiz) was the key to the beginning of everything!

I learned the importance of Community Service – the best gift you can give someone is your time. I became an active member of Delta Sigma Theta Sorority, Inc – a private, not-for-profit organization whose purpose is to provide assistance and support through established programs in local communities throughout the world. Delta Sigma Theta Sorority, Inc. provides an extensive array of public service initiatives through its Five-Point Programmatic Thrust of: Educational Development, Economic Development, International Awareness and

Involvement, Physical and Mental Awareness, and Political Awareness and Involvement.

Find something you are passionate about. Find others who are passionate about the same things. Become part of the group, the movement – it will be transformational!

Give Back! Always! My husband (Dr. Chiji Ohayia - Chief Ikukundu 1 (Ikukundu means "Breeze of Life")) and I have been sharing our blessings with the people of Eziachi Village in IMO State, Nigeria for many years, through our sponsorship of Medical Missions *once per year* and the installation of bore holes in compounds, enabling people to have immediate access to clean running water, reducing time and stress to travel to the stream. These activities will keep you socially connected. Connected to family, to friends deserving of you, to communities far and near and most, of all, to yourself!

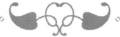

You can make a shattered glass impact.

You have unique skills and talents
to share with the world.

Please get to it!

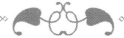

Here are some Social Wellness tips for you…

Humility is a good thing to practice.

Humility and peace go hand in hand. The less compelled you are to try to prove yourself to others, the easier it is to feel peaceful inside. Proving yourself is a dangerous trap. It takes an enormous amount of energy to be continually pointing out your accomplishments, bragging, or trying to convince others how great you are.

Here is a suggestion to develop genuine humility, *Practice*. By practicing, you will get immediate inner feedback in the way of calm, easy feelings. The next time you have an opportunity to brag, resist the temptation, STOP, listen to the little voice in your head – "Stop Don't Do It".

Tell at least one person, something you like, admire, or appreciate about them.

How often do you take the time to tell people how much you like, admire, or appreciate them? For many people it is not enough. Letting someone know how you feel about them - also feels good for the person offering the compliment. It is a gesture of loving kindness and means that your thoughts are geared towards what is right with someone. When your thoughts are geared in a positive direction, your feelings are peaceful.

Travel.

The world is a beautiful place with 196 countries to explore. Here are four proven health benefits of travel stated by The Huffington Post - Stress reduction, Heart disease prevention, Improved productivity, and Better sleep. My husband and I love to travel, during 2020 we planned to explore China and cruise the Mediterranean, however COVID-19 truncated our travel plans. Better to be healthy and safe than sorry. God willing, we will be able to fulfill our wanderlust cravings soon enough – until then we will be patient. Review and revise your "bucket list." Peruse the Internet for vacation and educational packages. Make tentative plans for the excursions you have always wanted to take and places you have always wanted to visit.

Volunteer.

The good we do have a way of boomeranging back to us. Volunteering can give you a sense of purpose, make your life more meaningful, increase your self-esteem, and make you happier. The greatest gift is to give our time to someone else.

Check out dog parks.

Many areas have dog parks – a great place to meet other people and socialize while your dog gets exercise.

Develop your own acts of kindness.

If you want your life to stand for peace, it is helpful to do kind and peaceful things. Acts of kindness can be defined as opportunities to be of service to others that are reminders of how good it feels to be kind and helpful. Here are a couple of examples, you might like holding the door open for people, visiting lonely people in a nursing home, or paying for the persons order behind you in a drive thru. The point is to think of something that seems effortless yet helpful to others. You will see, it is fun, personally rewarding, and produces a multi-faceted win for all parties involved.

Spend time with true friends.

How do you tell the real friends from the faux ones? The real friends like you for *who* you are, not for *what* you are or *what* you do. The best things in life are those things we can share with someone else.

Give compliments.

Everyone wants to be acknowledged. Everyone wants to be appreciated. A compliment costs nothing and will be remembered with a smile.

Explore someone else's world.

Have you ever stopped to think how little you know about the people you are around all the time, outside your immediate family? Ask questions, as this is a good way to understand a person. It can also help make you a better friend.

SURPRISE!

Most people like pleasant surprises. Why, because it means someone, or several people, care about and for us, that someone that has gone the extra mile, spent their time and energy, to plan and execute the surprise. The reward is making the other person feel better and seeing the smile on the other persons face.

Assess your relationship.

You have two (2) buckets:

1) Positive Relationship bucket: where there is mutual support with minimal stress. People that make "positive" or deposits to your emotional bucket. Your "true" friends are non-competitive with you, provide you with praise, and also "check" you when you are out of proper character.
2) Negative Relationship bucket: this is easy, as it is the complete opposite of the above. Everyone else that is not placed in the positive bucket. When you are around these folks, take your deep breaths, remember this too shall pass, and always wear a smile on your face.

Connect with people.

Pick up the phone and call friends, family, and customers you've neglected.

Thank you.

Saying Thank you is *free*. Write letters, emails, or a text to everyone who you owe a "thank you" such as co-workers, classmates, teammates, teachers, coaches and mentors. These two small words reveal sincerity, sensitivity, awareness, manners, and an overall approach to life.

Define your purpose; Define your mission (this may take a while).

Your purpose is your personal mission statement; it's how you plan to make your mark in this world. It will drive your decisions, strengthen your relationships, and steer you towards greater happiness and success.

My process began when I was laid off in 2005 and solidified in 2017, finally, putting all the pieces together, the birth of The Dr. Joy Brand Mission: "To Disseminate Relevant Wellness Information to Positively Impact the Lives of Others."

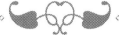

What is the reason for
your existence?

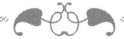

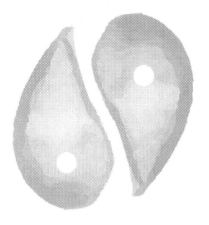

CHAPTER 5

Intellectual Wellness

Intellectual wellness refers to active participation in scholastic, cultural, and community activities. It is important to gain and maintain intellectual wellness because it expands knowledge and skills in order to live a stimulating, successful life.

My Story…

If you don't use it, you will lose it! Your ability to think that is! Your brainpower is muscle-memory, like any muscle, it needs to be exercised each and every day.

I am never bored. I do not have time for it! Back in 1993, I was introduced to my favorite game Mahjong, an Asian tile game played in the movie "Crazy Rich Asians". Four women in the neighborhood would get together every Friday evening for a few hours to engage in several hands of mahjong. There was more than mahjong going on – we were bonding, learning and testing our ability to create winning hands all the while talking, laughing, eating, etc. It is truly mental acrobatics and so much fun!

My husband gifted me a set, back in 1994. I instantly caught on to the rules and building hands with the various tiles presented. My math skills came in handy, as I would attempt to build multiple hands simultaneously until one would prevail. Hey, it's much harder than it sounds. My favorite hands are the Winds. I absolutely relish the opportunity to play a hand or two. Each year new cards are issued with new hands which require new strategies – hey, mahjong is not for the faint of heart! I always look forward to viewing the new cards published in April of each year. Oh, and did I mention – the high stakes? Yes, we gamble $0.25 per game. We are such big spenders!

With the proliferation of Apps, there are a plethora of games online. I have two favorite online games, solitaire and 2048. Don't laugh – I enjoy word find puzzles also.

Hey, I love anything numerical and credit my interest to my Father. He sparked my fascination with numbers and guess what? Years later I would earn two degrees in Applied Math and Statistics. These degrees really came in handy during my mahjong games – but, shhh, don't tell anyone I had a secret advantage!

My Mother is a living example of the importance of keeping your brain active at any and every age. Mom is a retired Registered Nurse (RN), whom, in 2020 at the young age of 88, still completes her "memory exercises" *as she calls them* daily to keep her mind sharp and dynamic.

Some of the exercises she favors are: Word Find, Duplicate Bridge, 500 Rummy, and Solitaire. Yes, she enjoys card games. During our visits together we play endless games of 500 Rummy. There is a snowballs chance in hell for me to ever have a winning streak as she wins the majority of the time, because she memorizes all of the cards that have been played! Imagine that! My Mother also enjoys assembling 500-piece puzzles. These are some of her exercises just to name a few. Oh, I forgot to mention my Mother is a member of a drama group, that's right she performs various short plays on stage a few times per year requiring her to memorize the lines for her character.

Here is a funny story. Mom and I love to bake sweet potato pies for the Winter holidays. As we gather all of the ingredients, when it comes to sugar, my Mother will recall and state the molecular formula for table sugar "$C_{12} H_{22} O_{11}$"! That's just one formula, she has others memorized and shares them if relevant during our conversations. Nevertheless, Chemistry was not my strong subject. But keeping a vigorous mind has become one of my passions as well. Thanks to Mom!

Another way to keep your mind sharp is by embarking on projects both short and long. Pick ones that are enjoyable and you will see, the time will fly by and you will be very pleased with the end results. For large projects, I would mind map all the elements to create the process. *What, wait – what is a mind map?*

Please tell me you're kidding – but here goes: A mind map is a diagram for representing tasks, words, concepts, or items linked to and arranged around a central concept or subject using a non-linear graphical layout that allows the user to build an intuitive framework around a central concept. Huh? Yep, and it's great for memory and brain dexterity! So just do it!

My goal is to learn something (anything new) every day. I read lots of articles and books, listen to podcasts and Thank goodness for Google. *Research* should be my middle name.

My girlfriends/BFFs from college (Stony Brook University) whom I have known since 1980, started our book club years ago as a way to stay connected. We discuss key learnings from each reading. Each month a new person will recommend a fiction or non-fiction book for us to read for the month. Usually, I am the one facilitating the book club discussion, maybe it's the television show producer and host in me. Oh, okay, you're right maybe I am just a little bossy too.

Learning new languages really challenge and strengthen the mind. Chiji and I are studying Mandarin Chinese, in preparation for our future excursion to China. We were scheduled to travel in May 2020, however COVID derailed our travel plans. But hey, there is a silver lining – we have more time to practice and master the language. Our brain neuron pathways thank us!

Please exercise and take care of your brain. Keep it healthy and strong. Memory and keen intellect do not have to diminish as we age. Staying mentally astute and productive really are keys to living a fulfilling, productive life!

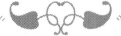

Remember, if you don't use
it, you will lose it!

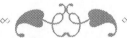

Here are some Intellectual Wellness tips for you…

Want to increase your Intelligence Quotient (IQ)? Enhancing your brain's capacity to plan, reason, and solve problems is always a good thing.

Here are some tips to increase your IQ:

Read more books.

Have you ever noticed that practically everything you read justifies and reinforces your own opinions and views on life? Want to improve your intellect? If your answer is yes, then I will encourage you to read more books and stretch your mind to think about things you normally do not think about. Keeping in mind, you do not need to change your core beliefs or your deepest held positions – you are just expanding your mind and opening your heart to new ideas. This new openness will reduce the stress it takes to keep other points of view away – as a result, you will see the innocence in others as well as increasing your patience.

I saw a sign in front of an elementary school which read "Reading is Like Dreaming with Your Eyes Open". Make reading and sharing thoughts fun and form a book club. I belong to a book club with two of my college friends. Although we are in different states, we discuss our thoughts via conference call or Face Time, one book each month. Our discussions are provoking, where everyone shares their point of view without judgment.

Read articles and books with entirely different points of view from your own and try to learn something.

Debate an issue with a friend.

But choose the viewpoint opposite the one you hold. Sounds tricky, right? That's the point! Focusing attention on information that is different than your beliefs can improve intellectual wellness. Naturally, we tend to only focus our attention on opinions, beliefs, and facts that hold true to our viewpoints. When you expose the mind to opposing ideas, it expands the mind to grasp new information. Here are two subjects to spark a conversation: politics and religion. Try it!

Learn something new each day.

Learn something new "every day" as learning is a continuous process. Learning new things about the way your mind processes information can be a vital tool to helping you succeed.

Set the resolution to learn something new every day in order to have a better understanding of the world and how it works.

Watch a TED Talk.

Watch a TED Talk every morning while you eat breakfast. My recent TEDx Talk is on ted.com and YouTube – *Are We Functioning Under Conflicting Knowledge Every Day?* Advice provided for a smooth divorce from internal conflict.

Pick up a hobby.

Did you know that having a hobby is good for you? Hobbies can lower your stress levels, boost your brainpower, offer a new challenge, improve your ability to focus, and promote staying present.

Learn a foreign language.

Learning a foreign language can be beneficial to your intellectual health and your employment prospects. When learning different ways to communicate, your mind expands. This not only helps with being receptive to new knowledge, but also helps broaden information already learned. My husband and I are learning to speak Mandarin Chinese, the most widely spoken native language in the world, yet the hardest language to learn due to the tonal nature of the language presents challenges at times.

Play a game.

Board games and cards are popularly known as leisure activities. These activities can also help with your intellectual wellness. The next time you have free time, pick up a deck of cards or pull out a board game and play – alone or with others. As long as your mind is thinking, improvements are being made. Chess will also help improve your ability to make strategic decisions in life. BINGO, Bridge, Mahjong, Chess, Solitaire anyone?

Play a musical instrument.

Music has a powerful impact on our minds. Playing a musical instrument can increase intellectual wellness by learning how to create sounds, make patterns, and emote through music. Any instrument can work to increase intellectual wellness, so start today and take up a new hobby.

Expose your mind to deeper thinking.

Take the time to write down thoughts, identify your feelings and gain an increased understanding of yourself and your actions.

Puzzles.

Working a crossword, word find, and Sudoku puzzle by finding words in patterns uses a great amount of brainpower.

Improve your memory.

Do you have a deck of cards? If so, a common game to improve your memory is "Concentration". Get a deck of 52 cards, 54 if the jokers are counted. Lay the cards face down on a surface, mix the cards, and then flip two cards face up over each turn. The object of the game is to remember the placement of each card and turn over pairs of matching cards.

Watch movies with sub-titles.

Interested in learning about a different culture? Expand your knowledge and watch movies with sub-titles. Some of my favorite movies/series have been: Unorthodox, Money Heist, and Nollywood productions.

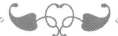

If you don't use it, you will lose it!

Your ability to think that is!

Your brainpower!

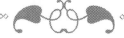

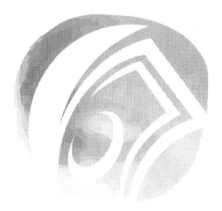

CHAPTER 6

Financial Wellness

Financial Wellness involves the process of learning how to successfully manage financial expenses. Money plays a critical role in our lives and not having enough of it impacts health as well as professional and academic performance. Financial wellbeing is about a sense of security and feeling as though you have enough money to meet your needs. It is about being in control of your day-to-day finances and having the financial freedom to make choices that allow you to enjoy life.

My Story…

Growing up, my mother ingrained in me some fundamental financial truths that have served me well over the years. Thank God I was smart enough to listen. Upon graduation from SUNY at Stony Brook, New York, I landed a job as a Statistical Engineer at Corning Glass Works. The first piece of advice from my mother to save 25% of each paycheck. WOW, that's a big chunk of change! Why did she tell me to do that? Because…drum roll, please! She wanted me to learn how to save for the future, since one way or another in LIFE, stuff happens! Okay, I thought, so I won't get that sports car! Another huge influence in my life came in the form of my husband, my partner in love for life even as ghosts! I wanted a big wedding, what girl doesn't? However, my soon-to-be husband pointed out that if we had a small destination wedding, we could use the money we would have spent on a larger wedding as a down payment on a home. It became the best decision we made at the time, besides getting married as it set us up financially. We were able to buy our first home just 10 months after we married! Not bad for a couple just 25 and 27 years of age! This was the start of us living with financial freedom! Over the years, many friends and some now non-friends have had the chutzpah (Jewish word for nerve, gall, tastelessness, and some other unprintable words as well, etc.) to ask us how we can afford our lifestyle. Really now!

Yet, in a way, I could understand. They saw a lifestyle in which I was downsized from corporate America, started an entrepreneurial endeavor and was still able to support two kids through private school. My answer to you (not them) is no secret: my husband and I achieved this through working smart and remaining focused. One of the biggest surprises I have found is when people let their talents or skills go to waste. Why would anyone give up on additional sources for income? For example, I utilized my two degrees in Statistics to communicate Math concepts effectively since I graduated college back in 1988 through private tutoring sessions, online and on-ground course delivery of undergraduate and graduate courses, and curriculum/course content development, for starters. My husband and I also invest in real estate outside of our primary home. These decisions allowed me to transition from corporate America to find, follow, and work my passion during my entrepreneurial journey, which began in July 2005.

Sounds like a fairy tale, doesn't it? I just laugh and laugh and laugh. Remember when my mother told me, "one way or another in LIFE, STUFF happens."! Yes, it does! And when it happens, it really happens! In my case, let's start with real estate investing. This was a decision I sort of convinced my husband to go along with me. In 2005, prior to my layoff, I became very greedy. Yes, me! We purchased a fully occupied commercial unit and several single units. *Note of consequence:* With real estate, the most important factor is location, location, location! Yet, we did NOT adhere to that rule as our investments were in a predominantly blue collar, distressed area. Nevertheless, I believed, incorrectly of course, that the income from the commercial unit would cover all expenses: mortgage, taxes, insurance, and extra money for ALL our investment properties! Ha! Did I learn a severe lesson here? You bet I did and here's what happened. We did NOT prepare for a recession! Surprise, Surprise! The second half of 2005 and 2006, we were cooking with gas! So, everything was going fine, we were collecting rents, all units were fully occupied and with minimal expenses for upkeep, maybe a broken toilet or two. We also had changed property managers, because our first one fired us when their focus shifted to large scale development projects, and guess what? We were too small for them!

We were still *Cinderella at the Ball,* even with these changes and did not see the evil stepmother approaching in the form of the aforesaid *Great Recession.* So, as soon as the clock struck 12:01am in 2007, we lost the proverbial *glass slipper* for the rest of 2007 and for years to come! We began to see a change with our revenue, our monthly checks received from our new property manager dwindled as the year progressed as there were late rents, vacancies and more expenses than we originally thought.

I am just warming up! Remember I had mentioned my entrepreneurial endeavor right after I was laid off from my corporate job in 2005. Well, I decided to become the owner, franchisee and operator of a Ladies Workout Express - Women's Only Health Club. Hey, I have been an award-winning runner all my life, so what could possibly go wrong? Hmmm…everything! I purchased the turn-key profitable club from the previous owners in September 2005. The club remained very profitable until 2007. During the second quarter of 2007, I started see the revenue line was on a slow downward trend towards the break-even line. We were now deep in the recession. I needed to make a very hard decision about renewing the 5-year lease contract for the club location to begin January 2008. Oh, where are crystal balls when you need them? Long story short, per the recommendation of my accountant, my decision was to donate all equipment and close the club. Like with my mother years before, thank God, I was smart enough to listen. But the fairy godmother I so badly needed was nowhere to be found! I was assessed $40,000 by the commercial property consortium because the location was not returned to its original 'vanilla' state! Sleepless night after sleepless night, I lived the nightmare of where the hell, was I going to come up with an extra $40,000!? I hired an attorney to represent me *yes, more money* to try to reduce the exorbitant fees to $20,000. Like, it's already been stated, stuff happens!

On top of everything else, there was less than expected revenue received from the real estate investments. By 2008, our real estate investments had gone straight down the drain! At this point, we were dealing with many vacancies due to people losing their jobs from 2007 through 2011 as a result of the recession. So, again, we were forced to make more hard decisions regarding our spending to keep current with our expenses. We had tuition costs, mortgage payments for residential and investment properties, and enrichment programs for our youngest son.

We received written correspondence from our mortgage company, with the offer to restructure our loan. We were in great standing with long history of paying on time on all real estate loans. We had the option to get a lower rate, reduced monthly payments, it was music to our ears, until … there was a catch. The mortgage representative mentioned we would need to suspend making mortgage payments on *all* real estate properties for a minimum of 3 months as this would show we were desperate for help. Really? We just wanted our rate adjusted! Thinking strategically, we were not in a position to forgo our mortgage payments, as we desired to retain our good credit rating. This would have been a catastrophic move for our family. Suspending mortgage payments for more than 30 days even for one property would have had a negative effect on our credit. We would have been denied for a car loan, business financing, another mortgage, and as a co-signer on a college educational loan! We made the decision to keep current with our payments, as the alternative would have hindered our children from achieving their educational goals.

We had to make further decisions to hold off on *all* non-essential purchases. Dining out (no way), grown folk extra-curricular activities (not happening), extra pampering sessions (spas, facials, etc. hey, what are you smoking? – gone in a heartbeat), outside entertainment, retail shopping, excursions, buying coffee at Starbucks (we made it at home), seeing our friends for a restaurant meal, going to a Broadway performance, vacations…NO, NO, NO and NO! It was painful for me to say NO, but it was imperative for us to stick to managing priorities to get through these difficult times.

There was one particular decision that was even more painful than all the ones listed above. I had to return my leased vehicle early (inclusive of remaining payments) to cut down expenses in the short term. Ouch and another ouch; however, I am now able to see how incredibly important that decision was.

And then there was this…we used our one credit card sparingly – only for emergencies. We used cash for all purchases, if we did not have the cash, we did not buy the item. During this time, I had a sneaking suspicion that some wondered and wanted to ask – if we had filed for bankruptcy. The answer was NO, and it was only because we made the decisions to say NO early to non-essential purchases. However, I believe bankruptcy can be a useful tool, and if it is deemed best for your situation, then by all means, file. Do remember, your financial situation is YOUR business only!

This is how we stayed the course and finally, finally, finally, we saw a glimmer of light at the end of a long tunnel! From these really difficult times, out came some truly great lessons that I am proud to share with you.

To keep our finances healthy and continually enjoy passive income streams; my husband and I follow some simple rules. And, you can do it too!

We pay ourselves first before our expenses. Hey, we have to eat, right? We have done this since my first corporate job in 1986, post-graduation from graduate school – as a Statistical Engineer for Corning Glass Works. This is key, just close your eyes and do this - save 20-25% every pay period! Ouch! Trust me you will not miss the money upfront, but it will give you power and peaceful sleep when you need it. Invest in real estate as soon as you are able, no you do not have to become a land baron, but a primary residence and investment property are good rules of thumb! *Note of interest:* My mom has owned real estate since she was 21 years old since 1953. I know, pretty incredible, right? My husband and I purchased our first primary residence (townhome) in 1988 several years later in 1995, we secured our first investment property and have been in the real estate investment game ever since. The monthly real estate expenses (mortgage or rent) should be covered with just one income preferably the lesser amount and then bank the other. Yes, you can do this. You really, really can!

Diversify, diversify, diversify your investments: your regular savings or as I call it: *MAD* money, company sponsored savings plan such as a 401K with company match or as I call it *FREE* money, real estate and another investment account outside of the company savings plan! Seek outside professional help from a financial advisor or wealth manager. These professionals will guide you towards achieving your goals. Interesting note: we first met with our financial advisor back in 1989, through my parents. He has been managing our money since then and now he manages our sons' investments. Pretty amazing, right? Talk about a trusted professional…now go find one for yourself!

Finally, we are coming to my favorite part: bonuses! Yep, for those fortunate enough to receive a bonus, how great! Yet, you still have to save! Oh no, not again! Yes, again! In our home, there is a rule. Receive a bonus, you can spend 10% and guess what you do with the other

90%? Right again, the money goes straight into the bank! Trust me, this will come in handy.

Looking back over all that has transpired: the layoffs, the great recession, underperforming investment properties, etc., which really should have stopped our lifestyle – I say Thank God we made hard choices early and often. That money is what saved our lifestyle and our life! Thank God for the good times and the hard lessons we gained during the difficult ones!

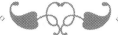

**Count your pennies and you won't
need to count your dollars.**

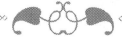

Here are some Financial Wellness tips for you…

Are you financially well?

A simple calculation will give you the answer. Have a sheet of paper and pencil or new spreadsheet, ready.

Are you living within or below your means? Do the following calculations to determine your answer:

a. Write down your annual gross revenue/salary from *all* streams of income at the top of the page. Yep, I said *all*...I hope you are not putting *all* of your eggs in one basket with that one gig.

b. Calculate 30% *your tax contribution* and subtract from your total gross revenue.

c. You have 70% remaining...sounds good? Now, take another 20% and designate this as your savings! Yes, your savings! You are going to save save save first...Always pay yourself first... remember this is about you!

d. The remaining amount is for your *expenses.*

Drum Roll Please...Are you able to cover *all* of your expenses with the last number on the page? If so, great! Congratulations! You are Financially Well!

If not, that's ok, you have some work to do and guess what, you can get started today! Here we go...this may be a sensitive subject, but it warrants some attention when it comes to *how* you spend your money.

Some practical tips to help you "Mind Your Money".

Are your friends making you overspend?

Are you trying to keep up with the Joneses? Do not act as though you have no idea about what you are reading here. Be honest with yourself. Do you want what your friends or neighbors have: The multiple luxury vacations, larger home, new car, planning an excessively expensive wedding, or any other material possessions? Let me just say this, and yes it is common sense: "Keeping Up with the Joneses can be very costly". It is better to *stay in YOUR own lane* and focus on your priorities! Be happy for your friends and more importantly, gracious for your situation, as "it" could always be worse.

A Harvard study conducted by Professor Nicholas Chritakis has shown that your friends can affect all of your habits including spending. His research shows that if you surround yourself with big spenders, you are more likely to spend, even though you know you should not. His research basically concludes – humans do not have the will power to control their lives. Do you really think this is the case? If so, we need to make a paradigm shift regarding spending habits. For additional information, check out this great book, *Connected: The Surprising Power of our Social Networks and How They Shape Our Lives,*

Live below your means.

Pay Yourself First - SAVE (there is that "S" word) 20% of your gross income. Overspending leads to stress. Stress prevents you from achieving total wellness – period end of story!

Set your priorities Needs vs Wants.

Needs first then wants. Create a "Wish" list for the items that you want and save small amounts towards those items, your list of "wants" will motivate you to stay on track.

Cut back on your expenses.

This is easy to accomplish especially if you pay cash for all purchases. yes cash…if you do not have the cash to for "IT", then do not buy "IT" until you do! Hey, that's how our family survived the recession that began in 2008.

Harness your skills.

A "side hustle" is a part time gig. You have many skills, do not let any go to waste! When you are busy, you do not have time to spend money and the added income from a second job can have a huge impact on your financial life.

Set clear family money rules.

For the parents out there, by saying "NO" and sticking to the family budget will teach your children about your family values and most importantly living below your means. I know this may be a challenge for some especially if/when your children will complain everyone else has "IT". For sure you as a parent will hear this comment from your kids. Check this out, to shut down the conversation, explain your reasons and Do Not Give In! Your children will eventually thank you later in life. My husband and I are proud parents of two grown independent sons, and this has worked for us.

Find a FBF (Financial Best Friend).

If you have a friend that is great at saving and without judgment, recruit them to be your FBF. The next time you feel the need to make a purchase, phone or text your FBF and ask them to help you stick to your budget.

Focus on the "plenty" in your life!

Remember those in need. Give what you can to help - your time will certainly make a positive difference.

Take charge of your finances.

Develop a plan to pay off debts, make a power payment on debts to reduce interest charges, and once that debt is cleared apply the payment amount to the next debt or save it!

Get your documents in order.

There are certain documents that every adult should have. According to Laurie and Yale Hauptman, partners at Hauptman & Hauptman, PC (previous guests on The Dr. Joy TV Show), start with "getting your paperwork" in order by creating your Estate Plan documents, which include but not limited to: your Letter of Instruction: Will or Trust and your Durable Power of Attorney. Without an Estate Plan, the government will decide how to split up your assets. Don't you think the government has enough control? Make sure the government does not have control over your assets. Take the necessary steps to create your Estate Plan, as it is an essential investment in protecting your assets.

To get started, feel free to contact Hauptman & Hauptman Law, Elder, Estate, and Special Needs Law www.hauptmanlaw.com. Reside outside the tri-state area of NY, NJ, and CT? Check out www.lawyer.com for legal professionals in your area.

Hire a professional.

Are you overwhelmed, yet? If so, you may need to hire a professional to assist you in getting your finances in order. Working with a financial planner can take the guesswork out of managing your money and help you make sound financial decisions. Talk to at least three planners to find the right fit. Having a professional to talk to about financial matters can ease your mind and reduce stress!

Practical tips to minimize your spending and stay on budget - Below are questions, I have answered during private sessions to help my clients pivot and make better financial choices to enhance their lives.

"I am living check-to-check, how do I assess my budget to see what is really going on?"

It is important to have a handle on where your money goes each month. There are many apps out there that will get all of your transactions in one place through technology, but I find it just as easy to pull up my checking account and credit card statements and write them all down. There is something magical that happens when you go through the exercise of writing down each expense. You create a true connection between your brain and your hand. Write down every transaction going back three months and dig in to find the random expenses that occur throughout that quarter. Then, create categories so you can see a full picture. Do not make this too complex. Five or six categories is plenty. Here are some examples: housing, food, entertainment, transportation, insurance and debt repayment for starters. Working through this process alone sheds light on where expenses can be reduced. Remember that even the smallest expense compounds over time, not just the amount, but the life of interest you could earn as passive income for not spending.

"I am very fortunate as I do not have any debt, however I want to save money. What are some smart ways to squeeze more from my paycheck?"

Pay yourself first. Send 15% of your pre-tax earnings to your retirement plan, and then into an investment account. If you have a few bucks, you really should find a professional advisor to help you achieve your financial goals.

"What are 3 ways to drastically cut my budget and reduce household expenses?"

Pretend as if you just had a child and one spouse quit working or just lost their job. At this time, you are forced to live on one income.

Sell a car, as a result, bye bye car note, automobile insurance, and maintenance. Do not worry, it is not the end of the world, when your situation improves, you will be in a position to acquire the current and enhanced model but for now, stick to the plan.

Stop dining out for a specified period of time, the money saved will add up quickly.

"Which are some painless ways to cut my expenses?"

o   Pack your lunch.
o   Cancel apps and subscriptions you pay for but do not use.
o   Cut your cable and use online streaming services.
o   Refinance any of your debt that makes sense, especially student loans and mortgages.

"What are two ways to have fun without the expense?"

Entertain on a budget. Once social distancing is no longer required, invite people to your house, have them bring a dish, their drink of choice, and watch a movie or play a game together. Rotate the venue each month.

Stay fit and have fun for a minimal cost. There are many great leagues for sports that do not cost a lot of money. Soccer, softball, kickball, and basketball all have great leagues in most cities and do not require thousands of dollars of equipment. They also take a couple hours out of your evening or weekend that might otherwise be spent at expensive happy hours or attending other entertainment events.

Write a business plan for your business...Your Career.

Do you have dreams of starting your business? Embarking on the entrepreneurial journey is not an easy feat. It can be done, with focus, tenacity, patience, and a solid business plan with actionable steps. A small business on the side? Ok, the first step to take is to write a business plan. Once you get your ideas down on paper, you will be that much more motivated to turn those ideas into reality. Even if you are working for someone else, have a plan of your own. Want to have a successful career? If your answer is yes, then make efforts to approach it as an entrepreneur, even if you are working for someone else. Think of your career as your own private business. I encourage you to market yourself, your abilities, and knowledge just as you would a product or service.

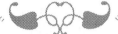

Plan today for a better tomorrow.

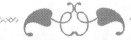

CHAPTER 7

Environmental Wellness

Environmental wellness inspires us to live a lifestyle that is respectful of our surroundings. This realm encourages us to live in harmony with the Earth by taking action to protect it. Environmental well-being promotes interaction with nature and your personal environment.

My Story…

While this wellness element may not seem to be as SEXY, it is just as important.

If there is one thing this pandemic has shown beyond a shadow of a doubt; it is our habits have damaged this beautiful planet. Now, I am not crying for the planet, oh no, with the world on quarantine, the skies are blue, the water is cleaner, the smog is lifting, Earth is thriving! It is so important to remember that the planet will go on long after we have destroyed ourselves with our sloppy and selfish habits. What habits am I talking about? So many, so little time, but let's get started. Can everyone say plastic?

I have detested plastic for a long time now and we are making strides to limit the use of plastic in our home. We store our foods in glass containers vs. plastic ones. Plastic straws, no way! My straws are stainless and I carry them with me and use them when I dine out. You think that's excessive! I will not use any plastic, plates, cutlery, anything!

Okay, got that out of my system! Moving forward, our home is a de-cluttered living space which means everything has its own place, you know, like we learned back in kindergarten. We do a *Spring* cleaning each May as well as a landscape cleanup outside. Yes, we declutter the closets too. Most people, including myself have clothes, shoes, accessories, etc. in the closet that no longer fit, either too big or too small. For those items, I have not worn in the last year or two, I ask myself, self… "Does this item bring me JOY?" If yes, I keep. If no out, out, out, it goes. Ahh, it really does make your body feel lighter and your brain clearer when you toss out the old, broken, damaged, etc., etc., etc.

Our household products are environmentally friendly "green clean" so I am keeping the environment as healthy as possible. I recycle weekly. Yes, we separate the garbage. We even rinse out our recycle bottles, cans, etc. We just do it! It's important! Would you like to know what we have done that is really easy and pays off big? We now have plants in our living space. Prior to COVID-19, we did not have any plants, but since March 2020, we have added plants in rooms where possible thus transforming a space suitable for quiet reading, yoga and meditation.

Interestingly, this one simple step has changed the entire landscape and feel of the room. Our air is clean, and it feels so good! Namaste!

Let's talk about energy levels and green living. On two occasions, I felt the need to raise the levels of positive energy in our home. What? Yes, we all need to be surrounded by positive energy and keep the negative energy at bay. Trust me on this one! We hired Dr. Michele Burgess a.k.a. Dr. B., of Wellness4Ever LLC. www.drbwellness4U.com, to incorporate Feng Shui principals to elevate the positive vibrations in our home. As we know from The Beach Boys, "Good Vibrations", are so important! Dr. B. traveled from North Carolina to New Jersey on two separate occasions to lend her expertise to rearrange and ground our home. It took some time to adjust to the changes, but within three months, we started to reap the benefits as positive vibes enveloped our living spaces.

We have removed the carpet from many rooms and replaced with hardwood, tile or marble. Okay, so not everyone was an early adopter! Years earlier, our sons begged us to keep the carpet in their rooms, which we did, to keep the peace, remember…we want positive energy. By the time you are reading this book, the carpet in their rooms should be gone, as a hardwood floor is so much cleaner and easier to maintain than a carpeted one.

We are non-smokers and we do not allow our guests to smoke inside or anywhere on our property. If you think it can't get much worse for our guests, then I have a surprise coming for you. We also request guests to rest their feet upon entering our home, but we are nice as we provide foot coverings so everyone can be comfortable and clean.

What else do we do to keep our home environment clean and positive? Well, many people have multiple televisions in their living spaces. We have one in the family room and none, not one, nada, in our bedroom, because the bedroom is for two things only *big HINT, they both begin with the letter 'S'*. Yes, the bedroom is for sleep and sex. Yes, I said it…sex, sex, sex…oh, grow up!

We have ceiling fans throughout our home. This conserves the use of our air conditioner (A/C) during the summer months. If the humidity is low, we open the windows and turn on the fans and it is so refreshing. If the humidity is high, well then, the A/C is on.

We replace the Allergen filters every 3 months; yep, that's once a quarter, nothing too drastic, right? Yes, right! Now, I have three more 'S' words coming your way. What? Oh, please get your mind out of the gutter – thank you very much! Our home utilizes septic for the sewer system. We have our tank cleaned every 2 and a half years like clockwork, in addition to regular maintenance inside the home. We are careful to only use *septic safe* toilet paper.

We are seriously considering a solar energy system for our home. Solar creates clean, renewable power from the sun and benefits the environment. This really does not seem too high a price to pay to keep our planet healthy, clean and green. Hey, We. Do. Not. Need. Another. Pandemic. To. Teach. Us. This. Lesson. Again. Are you all with me?

Save our planet.

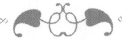

Here are some Environmental Wellness tips for you…

Your environment would include, your home, office space, car, furniture, clothing, airplane seat, and the list goes on and on…

Recycle.

Did you know recycling just 10 plastic bottles will save enough energy to power a laptop for more than 25 hours?

Did you know paper makes up nearly 30 percent of waste generated each year?

Did you know recycling one ton of aluminum cans conserves more than 1,204 gallons of gasoline?

Wait, did you know greasy pizza boxes are not recyclable? I bet many of you did not know that!

Here are a few tips on "how to recycle":

1) "Know what to throw" several containers are required for the following items:
    a. paper and cardboard - flattened cardboard, newspapers, magazines, office paper and common mail.
    b. metal cans – beverage and food cans
    c. plastic, and
    d. glass bottles and jars with lids. Check with your local area for specifics.
2) Keep all recyclables empty, clean and dry.
3) Do not mix items above.
4) Do not put recyclable items in bags.

For more information on "recycling" visit www.reuseplastics.org.

For my readers with a garden consider composting, reusing biodegradable waste, such as food or garden waste to help our environment.

Sanitize your surroundings with natural products.

Did you know the use of volatile plant oils, including essential oils, for psychological and physical well-being is the definition of aromatherapy, which dates back thousands of years? That's right, thousands of years ago it has been dated the Chinese and Egyptians were the first cultures to use aromatherapy with burning incense to create harmony and balance. There are over 100 essential oils that exist "the pure essence of a plant" that offer both psychological and physical benefits when used correctly and safely.

Here are my favorite three...

Lavender Oil.

Calming, alleviates stress, insomnia, and anxiety. There are clinical studies that support the use of lavender oil as an antiseptic. For additional information, check out https://www.ncbi.nlm.nih.gov/

Lemon Grass.

This oil is the one *bugs* hate. Lemon grass is used as a bug repellent. Place a couple of drops on a cotton ball and replenish your mind, body, and spirit. Place a few drops of your favorite citrus essential oil on a cotton ball and put in the refrigerator to help eliminate odors.

Tea Tree Oil.

This is a medicine cabinet in a bottle. Beginning as an all-purpose cleaner, combine 2 teaspoons of tea tree oil in 2 cups of water in a spray bottle. A few drops added to each load of laundry leave your clothes smelling cleaner. To keep germs at bay, spray it on highchairs, car seats, and other high traffic spots.

Ditch those other products that contain chemicals and ingredients we cannot spell nor pronounce, that are harmful to our environment.

Guard against germs.

We need to always be prepared just in case of a pandemic such as COVID-19. Here are some basic items in addition to the natural cleaning products recommended to have on hand at *all* times:

Homemade hand sanitizer – 1 tablespoon rubbing alcohol, 2 teaspoons aloe vera gel, and 10 drops of your favorite essential oil – mix together.

> Face Masks
> Rubber gloves (lots)
> Paper towels
> Toilet paper
> Lemons – rub 1 teaspoon of fresh squeezed lemon juice on your hands
> Vodka - Eyebrows raised, do I have your attention? Yep, 60 % alcohol or 120 + proof will kill many germs and works in a pinch to keep wounds and even equipment clean from infection causing bacteria. Always have a stash and use as a disinfectant.

Plants, plants, and more plants.

Plants can help improve air quality inside the house, as they act like a natural air purifier absorbing harmful chemicals making us healthier. For my readers with a "brown thumb" such as myself, opposite of "green thumb", the following plants for removing formaldehyde, benzene, and carbon monoxide from the air are recommended for your environment (these plants are located throughout my home, plant placement is dependent on lighting requirements):

> Peace Lily,
> Ficus Alii,
> Philodendron,
> Rubber Plant,

Bamboo Palm, and
Aloe. The aloe plant is multifaceted as it is used to treat skin conditions, such as psoriasis and acne Aloe creams have a calming effect on the skin and have been shown to help reduce itchiness and inflammation. Just break off a stem and use, simple as that.

Glass instead of plastic.

Do you remember back in 2010, the Food and Drug Administration (FDA) began warning about the harmful chemical bisphenol A (BPA) leaching into our meals when heated in a plastic container? For a peace of mind use glass as it is cleaner and safer than plastic. Glass containers are nonporous and will not absorb stains and the smell of the foods, perfect for storing hot and cold foods, including foods with intense color or smell.

Turn off your air conditioner.

Ok now, this is for everyone that uses the air conditioner. Most air conditioner recycle stale air. Just try this, if there is low humidity, turn off your air conditioner and open your window in the early morning, then shut the windows before the temperature rises by 9am. Use the ceiling fan for cross ventilation. As a result, you will enjoy fresh air inside and save on your utility bill.

Solar energy for your home or business.

Solar energy creates clean, renewable power from the sun and benefits the environment. Alternatives to fossil fuels reduce carbon footprint at home and abroad, reducing greenhouse gases around the globe. As electricity costs continue to increase, especially with longer and hotter summers predicted as our climate continues to warm, making the switch to solar the best way to lock in decades of predictable energy costs. Check out programs in your state to obtain incentives, rebates, and tax breaks.

Create your sanctuary to get a peaceful sleep.

First, as mentioned in the Physical Wellness Section, our body is like a battery; the only way to naturally recharge our body is to get enough rest. Your sleeping environment will have an impact on your sleep quality. Here are some tips to enhance your sleeping environment -

Let go of the television, computer or exercise equipment in your bedroom.

Too much technology will negatively impact the calmness within your space - so unplug and Let Go.

Have several levels of lighting in your bedroom or use a dimmer switch to adjust the energy accordingly.

Good, appropriate lighting is very important, as light is our # 1 nutrient and one of the strongest manifestation of energy. Candles are the best feng shui bedroom lighting, however, buy candles without toxins. Soy candles are recommended to achieve a nice calm light and use the soy to moisten your dry skin.

Use soothing colors to achieve a good feng shui balance in your bedroom.

Feng shui bedroom decor is a balanced decor that promotes the best flow of energy for restorative sleep, as well as sexual healing. Yes, I said sex! Best feng shui colors for the bedroom are considered the so-called "skin colors", and we know the colors of human skin vary from pale white to rich chocolate brown. Choose colors within this range that will work best for your bedroom decor.

Now follow the basic feng shui guidelines for your bed, which are:

- o   have your bed easily approachable from both sides,
- o   have two bedside tables (one on each side), and,
- o   avoid having the bed in a direct line with the door.

A "good looking" and well-balanced bed is very important in creating a perfect feng shui bedroom. Good mattress, solid headboard and good quality sheets from natural fibers are also very important in creating harmonious feng shui energy.

Keep all the bedroom doors closed at night, be it the closet doors, the ensuite bathroom door or the bedroom door.

This will allow for the best and most nourishing flow of energy to strengthen your health, as well as the health of your relationship.

Keep the toilet seat cover down ALWAYS!

The seat cover should always be put down before flushing, whether you are male or female, the entire discussion is moot. The reason that lid is there is to prevent what you are flushing from *spraying* into the room, which it does, no matter what is in the bowl.

Organized closet.

Keeping your bedroom closet clean and organized will further create a sense of peace and calm in your bedroom. Do you have trouble keeping your closet organized? If so, try this, on an inclement weekend make it a goal to clean out your closet. If it does not fit whether too small or too large, or you have not worn it in two years, put it in a pile, then donate to Good Will. There are many people that would be grateful to have your stuff. This will instantly increase your self-esteem as you have helped someone in need.

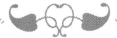

Make small changes to your environment
to positively enhance your health.

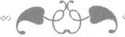

CHAPTER 8

Spiritual Wellness

Spiritual wellness is being connected to something greater than yourself and having a set of values, principles, morals and beliefs that provide a sense of purpose and meaning to life, then using those principles to guide your actions. Spiritual wellness provides us with systems of faith, beliefs, values, ethics, principles and morals. A healthy spiritual practice may include examples of volunteerism, social contributions, belonging to a group, fellowship, optimism, forgiveness and expressions of compassion.

My Story…

My transition to increase my Spiritual Wellness was in actuality a journey to match my deep belief in meaningful connection with someone or something bigger than myself. Lo and behold, this expedition aligned perfectly with my emotional health goals, thus creating a roadmap for finding and deepening my sense of overall Spiritual Wellness.

Born and raised as a Christian (Lutheran), I attended a parochial school for 13 years (K – 12 grade), the years seemed like a repetitive eternity, reading the bible, religion class, daily chapel service during school, and church service on Sundays.

Did I believe in a higher power? This was never a question for me. Yes, my higher power is GOD. What/Who is your higher power? You do not have to let me know now or ever, your choice think about it a bit.

Yet, as much as I was already a believer when the "not so good things did not go my way" as anyone alive knows too well, I would question God, why is this happening to me? With time, I began to answer my own question. Why not me? On numerous occasions, I may have wanted a certain thing or opportunity to happen only to find disappointment. God was probably laughing, the deep stomach-ache inducing type of laughter and saying "You are special. You need to learn some lessons, as lessons learned are actually blessings, and most of all you need to have patience." Patience, uh oh!

Things do happen for a reason. I seriously needed an attitude adjustment. Not my thinking at the time!

Life happens, some things we can prepare or prevent based on our decisions, but then there are those experiences of which we have NO control. Yes, those experiences… When this happens, we must let go of any false sense of control, we think or have thought we ever had and trust God or your higher power. Faith over Worry! Get rid of the negative thoughts and most of all have some patience. Again, with the patience, in God's time all will happen as it is supposed to.

In mid-October 2008, I was invited to join in an exercise of daily gratitude expression. Little did I know I was embarking on my transition to increase my spiritual and emotional wellness, pivoting to changing my thoughts, striving to be present and find JOY in the simplest smallest things. Someone may ask, what about the big things? Well, duh, that is obvious, we celebrate those too. Joy, your glass was always *full*. Can't you see?

During the time I started the exercise we were in the midst of the recession and the financial landscape for many was changing rapidly, present company included. However, I did not discuss or fight the challenges which, for controlish type of people like me, is SUPER hard. I just kept the faith and stayed on my grind. I am humbled and grateful for surviving the rough patch. Check this out, I believe the reason I was able to manage was because of the *change* in my attitude to include a bit of GRATITUDE! The act of scribing in my journal, positively changed my life. Wait, what journal are we talking about?

This is simple and here it goes. My friend suggested that I write down one reason everyday "Why I am Grateful" on a sheet of paper, notebook, journal, etc...So I began on October 15, 2008, 45 days before my 46th birthday scribing one reason of appreciation. The reason could be anything, something that may be small, or something that may be grand, the point is there was always something! These are your thoughts only, no one else. This is *all about you* on this very important life excursion!

This exercise has POSITIVELY changed my life as the focus was on the good things that happened during the day! Now, there is no need to go out and buy fancy journals or writing instruments, let's not complicate the process. I am sure all of you can find a spiral notebook for as little as $1 at the local grocery store. When traveling, my notebook is the first item packed in my carry-on bag, not my suitcase as it may get lost.

You don't know what to write about how you may feel? Oh, sure, you do! You absolutely do! Some of my previous entries included: remember this is only a few, I have been writing daily since October 15, 2008, you do the math, that is a lot of days - depending on the year you are reading this section it is for sure thousands of days and I never run out of things to include. Here is a sample of my entries:

- able to be grateful even in the midst of my own challenges,
- finding a parking space close to the store when I was in pain after surgery,
- when our son gained acceptance as a transfer student to his top college of his choice after a rejection the first go around. As a result, my blood pressure dropped back to normal range,
- to awaken and being able to breathe every day,
- being able to make someone else smile,
- solving a puzzle,
- having all my senses,
- weather: sun and rain,
- belly aching laughter,
- quality time with my family,
- protecting my children from harm,
- my own health and safety,
- day by day during my physical and mental/emotional healing journey in 2012 when each day was pretty bad as I kept questioning, why me? I was reminded and redirected...Why not me?,
- new experiences, different cultures, connecting with new people,
- rejections from directors and casting agents (NO = "New Opportunity"), you get the message...

I am always grateful for the *in your face* blessings and the covert lessons as hidden blessings we eventually discover later on.

Every year, on the day before my birthday, I review everything I have written over the past 365 days - my own self-reflective rite of passage, if you will. Can you guess what I have found? *Of course you can – but I'll say it anyway –* just noticing and practicing the rituals of gratitude leads directly to one big result! Say it with me – Increased Spiritual Growth! POW!

A huge thanks to Willa A. Edgerton-Chisler, MC, PCC Symphony Strategies div Symphony Coaching LLC, for urging me to begin my transformation process.

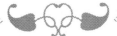

Happiness is not getting what you
want – It is enjoying what you have.

Here are some Spiritual Wellness tips for you...

Be more grateful and write it down daily.

Studies have shown that gratitude can make you 25% happier. Think about that for a second: you can be 25% happier simply by taking the time to count your blessings and think of all the good things in your life!

Being grateful will also help you to overcome adversity, improve the quality of your sleep, and allow you to get along better with others.

Remember *why* you are grateful. Record in your gratitude journal daily, as your situation can always be worse. Translating your thoughts into written words makes them more real.

Need a push to get started, not to worry…I've got you.

Here are the steps:

1) Get your notebook and pen;
2) Write todays date (first entry date) at the top of the page and inside the cover of the notebook;
3) Begin with the number 1 and begin writing – I Am Grateful to (fill in the blank – of *your higher power* and state the reason. One sentence that's it! No matter how big or small, there is no judgment, we all have something for which we are grateful. Should you feel the need to write more than one item per day, go for it! Remember to number your daily entries;
4) Write consistently at the same time during the day, perhaps take some time before you go to bed. Place the notebook and pen on your nightstand beside your lamp and clock;
5) Continue this for 28 days straight and it will become a habit;
6) Reflect every month, quarter and 364th day, as it will help you gain insight and see how to move forward.

Thank you.

Saying "Thank You" is free. These two small words reveal sincerity, sensitivity, awareness, manners, and an overall approach to life.

Pray and plank every day.

Mentioned in Chapter 3 - Physical Wellness, doing plank exercises every day is a great way to strengthen your core and express gratitude daily. Pray and plank demonstration during a Women's Empowerment Workshop.

Here are instructions on "how to" plank:

1) Find a space on the floor (a flat surface). Use a mat or towel for extra cushion if needed.
2) Lay flat on the floor.
3) Raise your body on your forearms and toes. Keep your head down.
4) First time planking, it is most important to hold and keep your balance.
5) Hold your plank for 1 minute (yes, set your timer).
6) Plank daily, increase time by 30 seconds, each month.

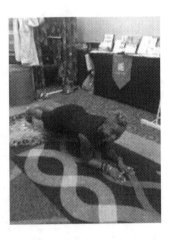

Forgive.

Carrying a grudge requires too much energy and keeps you in bondage, let IT go and free yourself.

More Faith less worry.

Five and 5, if it is not going to matter in 5 years, no need spending more than 5 minutes thinking about it.

Pick "one" word.

Select a word to guide you over the next 365 days. This word can be an anchor to help you set intentional goals and make decisions to improve your life. Three of my favorite guiding words thus far have been: Surrender, Impact, and Faith.

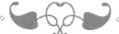

What is your "one" word?

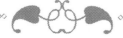

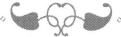

Messages to my younger self - 20's, 30's and 40's...

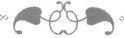

If I could go back in time, with my current knowledge, experiences, and increased maturity, here are messages to my younger self...

- **Have Patience.**
- When someone pays you a compliment and uses the words "cute" or "adorable", it is not a compliment. Excuse and ignore them, as they have a limited vocabulary.
- Money is not "everything", my health is paramount.
- Be like "Gumby", it is important to be flexible and adaptable to change.
- Spirit of Discernment – Always listen to your gut!
- Refrain from worrying as it is a wasted emotion.
- **Have Patience.**
- Everyone that smiles in your face and wants to share a meal is not your friend.
- Seek to understand others as this will eliminate judgment.
- Where you are at this moment is a point in time is not your destination in life.
- My thoughts matter, to me.
- Be "present" yet focus on the future simultaneously.
- Refrain from seeking validation from others.
- **Have Patience.**
- There is no need to compare yourself to others, as comparison is the root of unhappiness.
- No, does not mean NO, it means "New Opportunity".
- Keep your editorial thoughts to yourself.
- Live with purpose, each and every day. Even in a time of chaos!
- The ultimate "shoulder tap moment", use your crisis to reevaluate your life, pivot and make positive changes to move forward and keep it moving.
- Remain proactive about your happiness, not just reactive to the situation happening around you.
- **Have Patience.**
- Being "lazy" – is a good thing! Slowing down can actually be productive.

- Stop worrying about what it looks like on the outside and focus on how it feels on the inside.
- Don't sweat the small stuff.
- Live every day to the fullest.
- Be Present.
- If you do not ASK, you will not GET!
- **Have Patience.**
- God will work it OUT!
- Smile always and laugh often (this was tough during the first two years as an entrepreneur).
- It is OK to say NO and not be sorry!
- No Rules No Boundaries, especially in business.
- Be resilient.
- It is better to ask forgiveness than permission.
- **Have Patience.**
- Do not let toxic people rent space in your head.
- When someone lets you go, do not chase after them. Let them go.
- It is ok to LOVE from a distance.
- Mistakes are stepping-stones towards greatness.
- Learn from your mistakes. Find the lesson in each loss and Keep It Moving.
- Find your own path to fulfillment with enthusiasm and passion early. Become what you desire to become from your childhood dreams.
- **Have Patience.**
- Be vulnerable with people you trust.
- It's okay to have bad days and not hide them.
- It's okay to be less than perfect, as there is NO one perfect.
- It's okay to be yourself.
- Laugh at yourself.
- Be still, be quiet it will do you some good.
- **Have Patience.**
- You are enough!
- It's okay to do what is best for YOU.

- Asking for help is not a sign of weakness.
- Look for something positive in each day, even if you have to look a little harder.
- Friends and business do not mix, keep them separate.
- Do not obsess over what people think.
- **Have Patience.**
- There is always a solution.
- Notice what you do right on a daily basis.
- Challenges are put before you, to make you stronger.
- Run your own race.
- Praise yourself.
- Ultra self-critical tendencies must end.
- **Have Patience.**
- Success is defined when YOU can help others succeed.
- Empower and inspire others by sharing your story and experiences.
- You are: Exclusive, Extraordinary, Explosive, Inspirational, and Powerful.
- Progress outweighs perfection.
- Just when you think you have everything figured out, something else pops up requiring deeper thought. Do not rush the process.
- Stay in your lane and focus on your goals.
- **Have Patience.**

Simple, short advice
to my older self…

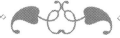

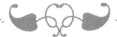

Have NO regrets,

Stay in the present,

Do whatever brings you JOY!

Question for you: What Brings You JOY?

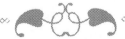

Recommended Resources

Websites:

Association For Applied Therapeutic Humor - https://www.aath.org/

Centers for Disease Control and Prevention - https://www.cdc.gov/

Connected the Book - http://connectedthebook.com/

Crash Course - https://www.thecrashcourse.com/

Dr. Joy Website – www.drxjoy.com

Eye Health - https://openyoureyes2020.com/

From Single Use to Reuse - https://www.reuseplastics.org/

Holistic Health Coaching - www.drbwellness4U.com

Huffington Post - https://www.huffpost.com/

Johns Hopkins Medicine - https://www.hopkinsmedicine.org/

Lawyer and Law Firm Directory - https://www.lawyer.com/

LifeStraw Products - https://www.lifestraw.com/

Men's Health - Fitness, Nutrition, Health, Sex, Style & Weight Loss Tips for Men - https://www.menshealth.com/

National Institutes of Health - https://www.nih.gov/

Positive Psychology - https://positivepsychology.com/

TED: Ideas Worth Spreading - https://www.ted.com/

Previously aired TV episodes of "The Dr. Joy Show – Your Prescription For Total Wellness" - https://vimeo.com/channels/drjoy

Women's Health - Fitness, Nutrition, Health, Sex, Style & Weight Loss Tips for Women - https://www.womenshealthmag.com/

World Health Organization - https://www.who.int/

Published Works:

Ohayia, Joy. *Don't Let IT Get You! An Empowering Health and Fitness Guide For Women,* Nebraska: iUniverse Publishing, 2007

Ohayia, J & Moore, G., *Are We Functioning Under Conflicting Knowledge Every Day?,* USA: Amazon-KDP Publishing, 2017

Ruiz, Don Miguel. *The Four Agreements: A Practical Guide to Personal Freedom (A Toltec Wisdom Book),* USA: Amber-Allen Publishing, 1997

Glossary of Terms

Balance comes in physical forms, emotional forms, and a spiritual form. For me, having a balanced life means creating time for the things I have to do, as well as the things I like to do.

Environmental wellness inspires us to live a lifestyle that is respectful of our surroundings. This realm encourages us to live in harmony with the Earth by taking action to protect it. Environmental well-being promotes interaction with nature and your personal environment.

Financial Wellness involves the process of learning how to successfully manage financial expenses. Money plays a critical role in our lives and not having enough of it impacts health as well as academic performance. Financial wellbeing is about a sense of security and feeling as though you have enough money to meet your needs. It's about being in control of your day-to-day finances and having the financial freedom to make choices that allow you to enjoy life.

Holistic Health is an approach to life. Rather than focusing on illness or specific parts of the body, this ancient approach to health considers the whole person and how he or she interacts with his or her environment.

Intellectual wellness refers to active participation in scholastic, cultural, and community activities. It is important to gain and maintain intellectual wellness because it expands knowledge and skills in order to live a stimulating, successful life.

Mental/Emotional Wellness, according to the World Health Organization, is defined as "a state of well-being in which the individual realizes his or her own abilities, can cope with the normal stresses of life, can work productively and fruitfully, and is able to make a contribution to his or her community." Emotional wellness inspires self-care, relaxation, stress reduction and the development of inner strength.

Nutritional Wellness is an in-depth study of the nutrients our bodies need and how we can best provide those nutrients for optimal health and wellness. The course looks at government regulations regarding the safety of our food supply as well as technology in food production such as genetic modification.

Physical wellness is the ability to maintain a healthy quality of life that allows us to get the most out of our daily activities without undue fatigue or physical stress. Physical wellness promotes proper care of our bodies for optimal health and functioning. There are many elements of physical wellness that all must be cared for together. Overall physical wellness encourages the balance of physical activity, nutrition and mental well-being to keep your body in top condition.

Social wellness refers to the relationships we have and how we interact with others. Our relationships can offer support during difficult times. Social wellness involves building healthy, nurturing and supportive relationships as well as fostering a genuine connection with those around you.

Spiritual wellness is being connected to something greater than yourself and having a set of values, principles, morals and beliefs that provide a sense of purpose and meaning to life, then using those principles to guide your actions. Spiritual wellness provides us with systems of faith, beliefs, values, ethics, principles and morals. A healthy spiritual practice may include examples of volunteerism, social contributions, belonging to a group, fellowship, optimism, forgiveness and expressions of compassion.

Wellness is an active process of becoming aware of and making choices toward a healthy and fulfilling life.

About the Author

Dr. Joy Ohayia, extremely passionate about health and wellness in all aspects of her life, strives to bring that same enthusiasm to others.

The Dr. Joy Brand Mission: "To Disseminate Relevant Wellness Information to Positively Impact the Lives of Others."

Dr. Joy is the host of the award-winning local cable TV Show, The *Dr. Joy Show – "Your Prescription For Total Wellness"*. The show has a focus on "The Seven Elements of Total Wellness," comprising of physical, nutritional, social, environmental, financial, spiritual, and mental/emotional aspects.

Dr. Joy is a highly sought-after motivational speaker and author of several published works including: *Are We Functioning Under Conflicting Knowledge Every Day?*, *Don't Let "IT" Get You!: An Empowering Health and Fitness Guide for Women*. In addition, Dr. Joy is featured in *"Blueprint for Success - Proven Strategies for Success and Survival,"* alongside Stephen Covey and Ken Blanchard.

Fortune 500 companies have also benefited from Dr. Joy's proven strategies for success, through a program tailored to meet the specific needs of companies and its employees. Healthy, Wealthy and Wise: *"Your health is your wealth. Healthy employees make a wealthy company."*, is the mantra of The Dr. Joy Workplace Wellness Program, which addresses mental, emotional, and social factors through customized programming.

She holds a PhD in Natural Health and Holistic Nutrition and Healing from the University of Natural Health, Master of Science, and Bachelor of Science degrees in Applied Math and Statistics, from

Rutgers University and Stony Brook University, respectively. During her tenure at Stony Brook University, Joy (Enoch), achieved numerous accomplishments in the sport of Track and Field, earning four individual records for sprinting, one of which still remains unbroken since 1984. She is a nationally ranked sprinter with the master's division of the USATF (USA Track and Field).

Dr. Joy Ohayia received international award recognition as the "2017 Disruptor of The Year" presented by Whole Life Activation based in the UK, an organization that celebrates the achievements of phenomenal women across the globe.

She also served two terms as a Board Trustee for the State of New Jersey chapter of CASA, a children's advocacy group.

Dr. Joy and her husband, Chiji have been married since 1987. They are grateful for their health, while laughing and enjoying life together every day.